SIRTFOOD DIET COOKBOOK

Healthy Sirtfood Diet Recipes to Use in Your Meal Plan

(The Complete Beginner's Cookbook to Unlock Your Metabolism)

Roland Molina

Published by Alex Howard

Sirtfood Diet Cookbook: Healthy Sirtfood Diet Recipes to Use in Your Meal Plan (The Complete Beginner's Cookbook to Unlock Your Metabolism)

ISBN 978-1-77485-014-5

Legal & Disclaimer

The information contained in this book is not designed to replace or take the place of any form of medicine or professional medical advice. The information in this book has been provided for educational and entertainment purposes only.

Table of contents

Part 1

Introduction

The main scientific evidence supporting this diet was the discovery that sirtfoods are found in the diet of people with the lowest incidence of disease and obesity rates in the world, such as the American Kuna Indians or the Japanese of Okinawa.

However, much of the weight lost comes, not exactly from the food eaten, but from the drastic cut in energy value, particularly in the first phase. Due to the restriction and the juice-based diet, the loss of water and even loss of muscle mass causes the values on the scale to decrease substantially.

In addition, the studies were carried out in people whose physical activity is high, an activity that, in itself, activates the "lean genes" and contributes to the increase in longevity.

The traditional Mediterranean diet is the one that brings together the most consensus for weight loss and health improvement, being a dietary pattern that includes several sirtfoods, such as virgin olive oil or red wine, fruit, vegetables, among others that contain vitamins and antioxidants.

IN SHORT...

It is useful to know the sirtfoods that activate sirtuin since they are healthy foods and rich in antioxidants, which enhance health and can stimulate basal metabolism.

However, the majority of weight loss will be derived from the promoted energy restriction, which is the main factor for weight loss in any diet.

The Sirtfood diet is rich in healthy foods, but not healthy eating patterns. In addition to promoting rapid weight loss without elucidating what is being lost, quite serious health claims are made without any scientific evidence to support them.

Adding SIRT-rich foods to the food day is not at all a bad idea and can bring health benefits, but this is just another restrictive diet like so many others, with nothing special worth the buzz created around it.

Who is the diet suitable for?

The Sirtfood Diet is suitable for:

People with perseverance and discipline

nutrition-loving people with background knowledge

The Sirtfood Diet is not suitable for:

People who have a hard time consuming only a few calories every day

Smart tips for everyday life

Many advisers reveal which other foods are suitable for the sirtfood diet and which other foods are combined with them. These can be helpful in order to plan daily food preparation better and thus make it easier. Because a comprehensive knowledge of sirtuins, their effects and how to best integrate them into your daily diet increases your stamina.

Relaxation is also an essential part of the sirtfood diet. In stressful situations, the hormone cortisol is released, which, together with insulin, stimulates blood sugar levels and causes the body to feel hungry during periods of rest. Mainly due to the calorie reduction, one should avoid stressful situations in everyday life as much as possible. Small activities to balance out like a little walk in the fresh air can work wonders.

Given that this has just reached mainstream awareness over the past year, you will be forgiven not to learn what the 'Sirtfood Diet' is. However, the diet has grown in both prominence and reputation after a number of celebrity endorsements, also encroaching on the 'Keto' diet and related Duran diet. The diet has been famous most recently after Adele was confirmed to have adopted it, contributing to a substantial weight loss.

If you adopt the diet closely, you will lose weight. If you are eating 1,000 calories of tacos, 1,000 calories of kale, or 1,000 calories of snickerdoodles, at 1,000 calories, you can lose weight. But she also points out that, with a more rational calorie limit, you will have results. The average regular consumption of calories by those not on a diet is 2,000 to 2,200 but decreasing to 1,500 is also limiting and should be a successful weight-loss method for others.

Chapter 1: What Are Its Basic Principles And What Is Its Purpose?

Sirtuins are a group of proteins that manage cell wellbeing. Sirtuins assume a key job in controlling cell homeostasis.

In the workplace, there are numerous individuals taking a shot at different assignments with an extreme objective: remain gainful and satisfy the strategic the organization in a productive way for whatever length of time that conceivable. In the cells, there are numerous pieces taking a shot at different undertakings with an extreme objective, as well: remain sound and capacity proficiently for whatever length of time that conceivable. Similarly, as needs in the organization change, because of different inside and outer variables, so do needs in the cells. Somebody needs to run the workplace, directing what completes when, who will do it and when to switch course.

NAD+ is essential to cell digestion and many other organic procedures. In the event that sirtuins are an organization's CEO, at that point, NAD+ is the cash that pays the pay of the CEO and workers, all while keeping the lights on and the workplace space lease paid. An organization, and the body, can't work without it.

Protein may seem like dietary protein — what's found in beans and meats and well, protein shakes — yet for this situation we're discussing atoms called proteins, which work all through the body's phones in various capacities. Consider proteins the divisions at an organization, everyone concentrating without anyone else explicit capacity while planning with different offices.

Acetyl bunches control explicit responses. They're physical labels on proteins that different proteins perceive will respond with them. In the event that proteins are the branches of the cell and DNA is the CEO, the acetyl bunches are the accessibility status of every division head. For instance, in the event that a protein is accessible, at that point the sirtuin can work with it to get something going, similarly as the CEO can work with an accessible division head to get something going.

Sirtuins work with acetyl bunches by doing what's called deacetylation. One way that sirtuins work is by evacuating acetyl gatherings deacetylating organic proteins, for example, histones. The histone is an enormous cumbersome protein that the DNA folds itself over. This loosened up chromatin implies the DNA is being translated, a fundamental procedure.

We've just thought about sirtuins for around 20 years, and their essential capacity was found during the 1990s. From that point forward, specialists have rushed to examine them, recognizing their significance while likewise bringing up issues about what else we can find out about them.

In 1991, Elysium fellow benefactor and MIT scientist Leonard Guarente, close by graduate understudies Nick Austriaco and Brian Kennedy, directed tests to all the more likely see how yeast matured. By some coincidence, Austriaco attempted to develop societies of different yeast strains from tests he had put away in his ice chest for quite a long time, which made an unpleasant situation for the strains.

This is the place acetyl bunches become possibly the most important factor. It was at first idea that SIR2 may be a deacetylating protein — which means it expelled those acetyl gatherings — from different atoms, however, nobody knew whether this was valid since all endeavors to show this movement in a test tube demonstrated negative.

In Guarente's very own words: "Without NAD+, SIR2 sits idle. That was the basic finding on the circular segment of sirtuin science."

Ecological factors significantly influence the destiny of living beings and sustenance is one of the most persuasive variables. These days life span is a significant objective of medicinal science and has consistently been a fabrication for the individual since antiquated occasions. Specifically, endeavors are planned for accomplishing effective maturing, to be specific a long life without genuine ailments, with a decent degree of physical and mental autonomy and satisfactory social connections.

Gathering information unmistakably exhibits that it is conceivable to impact the indications of maturing. Without a doubt, wholesome mediations can advance wellbeing and life span. A tribute must be given to Ancel Keys, who was the first to give strong logical proof about the job of sustenance in the wellbeing/sickness balance at the populace level, explicitly in connection to cardiovascular illness, still the main source of death overall. It is commonly valued that the sort of diet can significantly impact the quality and amount of life and the Mediterranean eating regimen is paradigmatic of an advantageous dietary example The developing cognizance of the useful impacts of a particular dietary example on wellbeing and life span in the second 50% of the only remaining century produced a ground-breaking push toward structuring eats fewer carbs that could diminish the danger of constant maladies, subsequently bringing about solid maturing. Subsequently, during the 1990s the Dietary Approaches to Stop Hypertension Dash diet was contrived so as to assess whether it was conceivable to treat hypertension not pharmacologically. To be sure, the DASH diet was very like the Mediterranean Diet, being wealthy in foods grown from the ground, entire grains, and strands, while poor in creature-soaked fats and cholesterol. The awesome news leaving the investigation was that not exclusively did the DASH diet lower circulatory strain, however, it additionally diminished the danger of cardiovascular infection, type 2 diabetes, a few sorts of malignant growth, and other maturing related maladies To improve the medical advantages

7

of plant nourishment rich additionally, creature fat-terrible eating routines, especially in hypercholesterolemic people, the Portfolio Diet was planned This eating regimen, other than being to a great extent veggie-lover, with just limited quantities of soaked fats, prescribes likewise a high admission of utilitarian nourishments, including thick filaments, plant stanols, soy proteins, and almonds. Curiously, members on the Portfolio Diet displayed a decrease of coronary illness chance related to lower plasma cholesterol and incendiary files in contrast with members on a sound, for the most part, vegan diet.

Nonetheless, additionally, the measure of ingested nourishment has been pulling in light of a legitimate concern for mainstream researchers as a potential modifier of the harmony among wellbeing and infection in a wide range of living species. Specifically, calorie limitation CR has been exhibited to be a rising healthful intercession that animates the counter maturing instruments in the body.

In this way, the eating routine of the individuals living on the Japanese island of Okinawa has been widely broken down on the grounds that these islanders are notable for their life span and expanded wellbeing range, bringing about the best recurrence of centenarians on the planet. Interestingly, the customary Okinawan diet came about to be fundamentally the same as the Mediterranean Diet and the DASH diet regarding nourishment types. Be that as it may, the vitality admission of Okinawans, at the hour of the underlying logical perceptions, was about 20% lower than the normal vitality admission of the Japanese, along these lines deciding an average state of CR.

 Singer Adele has confirmed that she has lost 30 kilos in just one year. The secret? Apparently, it's all thanks to the Sirtfood Diet. It was revealed by the singer herself through international media, such as the Daily Mail and the New York Post.

The Sirtfood Diet is not the classic fasting diet: Adele is the living proof of this, given the splendid shape in which was at her appointments with her fans. It is, in fact, a diet that leaves room for both cheese and red wine as well as chocolate, in the right proportions, and of course under the supervision of a specialist doctor, who knows how to evaluate your health and recommend the most suitable diet to lose weight safely.

Many were the media that underlined the substantial weight loss of the singer Adele who admitted, how the decision to lose weight did not depend on the acceptance of herself as much as the difficulty of using her voice to the fullest.

Adele praised the Sirtfood Diet, which made her lose 30 kilos without much effort although in reality, she admitted via Instagram that she had never struggled as much in physical activity as when preparing for her tour). She also said that the beauty of Sirtfoods is that many of them are already on our table every day. They are accessible and can be easily integrated into our diet.

Although being thinner was not her priority the singer has always had an excellent relationship with her body), she wanted to check her eating habits to get back in shape, but also or better above all to feel good about herself.

Furthermore, the Sirtfood Diet had come back on the news because it was Pippa Middleton's choice to get back into shape quickly before her wedding with the millionaire James Matthews that was celebrated on May 20, 2017.

Here are three motivations to take a pass on the sirtfood diet:

The sirtfood diet estimates achievement just as far as weight loss.

I've said it before and I'll state it once more: Weight is a determinant of wellbeing, yet it's not alone. To gauge somebody's wellbeing accomplishment on whether they lose X pounds in X measure of time overlooks the various advantages of nourishment. Nourishment is brimming with vitality, which enables you to do things like showering, practicing and relaxing.

It additionally has supplements that can advance a few substantial capacities and is often a cheerful encounter established in custom. For by and large wellbeing, there's a great deal more to concentrate on than basically appearance and estimating achievement just as far as weight loss is incomprehensive.

It's prohibitive, which can harm your association with nourishment.

This diet stresses an admission of 1,000 to 1,500 calories for every day, which is a lot of lower than a great many people need. When we seriously limit our nourishment admission, our intuitive response is to indulge. Your body is savvy, and it thinks about this absence of sustenance as an assault. Therefore, we will in general overcompensate, which is the reason we as a whole can identify with being "hangry" and thusly overindulging when we're at last allowed to eat. Rehearsing careful and instinctive eating is a more practical course than confining nourishment.

The sirtfood diet isn't science-based.

While there is some questionable research about the advantages of sirtuins, there's practically zero research about the specific sirtfood diet. Moreover, we as of now have a few rules set up that have been completely looked into and tried for quite a long time. If you're lost on what "sound nourishment" is, this is a superior spot to begin.

It's thoroughly fine if you need to join a couple sirtfoods into an eating plan. All things considered, nourishments like green tea, organic product, dim chocolate, and kale all include a spot inside a smart dieting design! Be that as it may, holding fast to a program with such exacting pass-or-bomb prerequisites is unreasonable and could be hurtful to your association with nourishment. By fusing an eating plan that is loaded with assortment and eating carefully, you'll have the option to set up a long haul, manageable association with nourishment. Cheers to that!

Chapter 2: How It Works And Its Effectiveness

Surely the diet will seem to work for certain individuals. In any case, scientific confirmation of any diet's triumphs is an altogether different issue. Obviously, the perfect investigation to think about the viability of a diet on weight loss (or some other result, for example, maturing) would require an adequately enormous example – delegate of the populace we are keen on – and irregular distribution to a treatment or control gathering. Results would then be checked over an enough timeframe with severe command over puzzling factors, for example, different practices that may decidedly or adversely influence the results of enthusiasm (smoking, for example, or work out).

This examination would be constrained by techniques, for example, self-revealing and memory, however, would go some approach to finding the viability of this diet. Research of this nature, be that as it may, doesn't exist and we ought to therefore be wary when deciphering essential science – all things considered, human cells in a tissue culture dish presumably respond differently to the phones in a living individual.

Further uncertainty is thrown over this diet when we think about a portion of the specific cases. Losses of seven pounds in a single week are ridiculous and are probably not going to reflect changes to muscle to fat ratio. For the initial three days, dieters expend around 1000 kcal every day – around 40–half of what a great many people require. This will bring about a fast loss of glycogen (a put away type of starch) from skeletal muscle and the liver.

Yet, for each gram of put away glycogen we additionally store roughly 2.7 grams of water, and water is overwhelming. So, for all the lost glycogen, we likewise lose going with water – and henceforth weight. Furthermore, diets that are too prohibitive are difficult to follow and bring about increments in hunger invigorating hormones, for example, ghrelin. Weight (glycogen and water) will therefore come back to typical if the desire to eat wins out.

As a rule, use of the scientific technique to the investigation of sustenance is difficult. It is often unrealistic to do fake treatment-controlled preliminaries with any level of natural legitimacy, and the wellbeing results that we are often keen on happen over numerous years, making research configuration testing. Besides, considers in huge populaces rely upon shockingly shortsighted and guileless information assortment strategies, for example, memory and self-announcing, which produce famously inconsistent information. Against this foundation commotion, nourishment look into has a difficult activity.

Is There A Quick Fix?

Sadly, not. Sensationalized features and often hyperbolic portrayal of scientific information brings about the apparently unlimited debates about what – and how much – we ought to eat, further fueling our fixation on a "convenient solution" or marvel fix, which in itself is an endemic social issue.

For the reasons sketched out, the Sirtfood diet ought to be entrusted to the prevailing fashion heap – at any rate from a scientific point of view. In light of the proof we have, to recommend in any case is, best case scenario fake and even under the least favorable conditions deceiving and harming to the authentic points of general wellbeing procedure. The diet is probably not going to offer any profit to populaces confronting a scourge of diabetes, sneaking in the shadow of corpulence. As expressed plainly by others, uncommon diets don't work and dieting all in all is certainly not a general wellbeing answer for social orders where the greater part of grown-ups are overweight.

By and by, the best technique is long haul conduct change joined with political and natural impact, focused on expanded physical movement and some type of cognizant command over what we eat. It is anything but a convenient solution, yet it will work.

A diet that underlines dull chocolate, red wine, kale, berries, and espresso? It either seems like the most ideal street to wellbeing and weight loss, or unrealistic. However, pause, it shows signs of improvement: According to the makers of the Sirtfood Diet, these and other supposed "sirtfoods" are indicated to enact the components constrained by your body's characteristic "thin qualities" to assist you with consuming fat and get more fit.

Bragging a rundown flavorful nourishment, you presumably as of now love, and supported by reports that Adele utilized it to get in shape in the wake of having a child, the Sirtfood Diet sounds naturally engaging.

Be that as it may, not to destroy your chocolate-and-red-wine high here, yet the science doesn't really bolster the diet's greatest cases. Which isn't to say that eating sirtfoods is an ill-conceived notion . . . yet, similarly as with all diets that sound unrealistic, you should take a gander at this one with genuine examination. This is what you have to think about what sirtfoods can and can't accomplish for you.

As a matter of first importance, what the hell is a sirtfood?

Manufactured by U.K. Sustainance experts Aidan Goggins and Glen Matten, the Sirtfood Diet highlights plant-based feeding stuffs known as "sirtuin activators." Basically, you animate the SIRT1 quality encoded proteins that Goggins and Matten called "thin quality" when you look at the key arrangement fixtures.

SIRT1 and sirtuin proteins are accepted to assume a job in maturing and life span, which might be identified with the defensive impacts of calorie limitation. The case behind the

14

Sirtfood Diet is that sure nourishments can actuate these sirt-intervened pathways sans the limitation, and consequently "switch on your muscle to fat ratio's consuming forces, supercharge weight loss, and assist fight with offing infection."

Alongside red wine, dull chocolate, berries, espresso, and kale, sirtuin-advancing nourishments incorporate matcha green tea, additional virgin olive oil, pecans, parsley, red onions, soy, and turmeric (a.k.a. phenomenal flavors and go-to solid treats).

There's some science behind the cases of sirtfoods' advantages, yet it's exceptionally constrained and rather disputable.

The science on the sirt boondocks is still very new. There are contemplates investigating the SIRT1 quality's job in maturing and life span, in maturing related weight addition and maturing related illness, and in shielding the heart from aggravation brought about by a high-fat diet. In any case, the examination is restricted to work done in test tubes and on mice, which isn't adequate proof to state that sirtuin-boosting nourishments can have weight loss or against maturing capacities in an absolutely real human body.

Brooke Alpert, R.D., creator of The Sugar Detox, says there's exploration to recommend that the weight-control advantages of sirtfoods may come to some degree from the polyphenol-cancer prevention agent resveratrol, often advertised as a component in red wine. "All things considered, it is difficult to devour enough red wine to get benefits," she says, noticing that she does much of the time recommend resveratrol enhancements to her customers.

Also, some nourishment specialists aren't psyched about the way the Sirtfood Diet plan works.

According to top dietitians who've evaluated the arrangement, the Sirtfood Diet is feeling the loss of some significant components for a sound, adjusted routine. Goggins and Matten's diet plan includes three stages: a couple of days at

1,000 calories for each day, made up of one sirtfood-overwhelming dinner and green squeezes; a couple of long periods of two sirtfood suppers and two squeezes per day, for an aggregate of 1,500 calories; and a fourteen day support period of sirt-y suppers and juices.

Keri Gans, R.D., creator of The Small Change Diet, says that she's "not wild about anything that runs in stages." Usually, the shorter stages make a hardship organize, which just prompts gorging eventually. "When you're limiting, anybody will get in shape toward the beginning of a diet," she clarifies. "However, we can't continue that eating design long haul."

According to Lauren Blake, R.D., a dietitian at the Ohio State University Wexner Medical Center, when you're hydrating and squeezing a great deal without a huge amount of calorie consumption, weight loss is normal, "however it's ordinarily liquid loss," she clarifies. So, while one may shed beats on the diet, it's probably going to be impermanent and might have nothing to do with sirtuins by any means.

The decision? Sirtfoods are incredible to have in your diet, however they shouldn't be all you have.

There's positively no explanation you can't include some sirtfoods into your eating plan, says Alpert. "I think there are some truly fascinating things here, similar to the red wine, dull chocolate, matcha—I love these things," she says. "I love mentioning to individuals what to concentrate on rather than what to nix from their diet." If it tastes liberal and it's solid in little amounts, why not?

Gans says she's an enthusiast of a ton of the nourishments on the sirt list, including staples of the Mediterranean Diet—the highest quality level of scientifically-supported smart dieting—like olive oil, berries, and red wine. "I can get behind nourishments rich in polyphenols and cancer prevention agents," she says.

Blake concurs that there's bounty to adore about the nourishments remembered for the diet, particularly the stylish fixings like turmeric and matcha that vibe crisp and help make eating fun and intriguing. "I'm seeing a great deal of plant-based nourishments that truly sparkle, and are loaded up with phytonutrients," she says. "Those are calming, and bravo."

Be that as it may, all the nourishment specialists recommend balancing the diet with some lean protein and sound fats, for example, progressively nuts and seeds, avocado, and greasy fish like salmon. Stir up your plate of mixed greens game, as well, with more kinds of veggies, spinach, and romaine lettuce notwithstanding the kale and red onions. Main concern? A large portion of the sirtfoods are An OK to eat and solid for you, yet simply don't depend on the diet to enact any "thin quality" right now.

Chapter 3: What Are The Foods That Regulate Biological Pathways?

Top 20 foods in the sirtfood diet:

The sirtfood diet comprises of a variety of different foods. The most significant benefit of a sirtfood diet is the wide variety of different food spectrum which can be incorporated in our personalized diet plan. The sirtfood diet can also have coffee and wine, which is the most popular reason that many celebrities are following this diet plan. sirtfoods are the most common and most widely used foods in both the Western and Eastern worlds. To be very specific, sirtfoods are those which contain high levels of a chemical compound called polyphenol. This compound is not uniformly distributed in sirtfoods, but every sirtfood contains specific amounts of polyphenols. You must be thinking that why only polyphenols are being tackled here. The answer is straightforward yet very informative. Polyphenols are the compounds that are present naturally in sirtfood, and many types of research conducted on these foods have confirmed that these foods have the highest impacts when losing extra pounds of fats from the body.

However, the most famous foods in the sirtfood diet are actually twenty in number, and a significant portion of a sirtfood diet comprises of these superfoods. The reason to stick this food on a more significant proportion of the sirtfood diet is the higher number of polyphenols present in these foods, which is essential to unlocking the sirtuin gene in the body. This gene is arguably the most critical gene to trigger many fat loss cycles in the human body.

The top twenty sirtfoods are:

Arugula:

The critical factor is the nutritious benefits provided by this food, which is rich in very unique and rare benefits. It is an outstanding food that can be used in health promotion and anti-aging. It is also called a superfood. A vast scientific literature is dedicated to supporting this food. It contains high amounts of antioxidants, antifungal, antiviral, disinfectant, and protecting benefits. It is also essential In the reduction of cholesterol from the body and thus reduces the chances of atherosclerosis and heart attacks.

A word Rasayana is used in traditional Indian medicine, which is associated with the global benefits of arugula in the human body. Arugula is a natural coolant that can be a protective remedy during hot summers. It also has cooling effects on the liver and stomach.

Buckwheat:

Stomach acids, disturbed gut mobility and injured food canal (esophagus) cause heartburn, a condition that affects every human many times in their lives. Buckwheat prevents heartburn by improving the capacities of the stomach and colon as well as by healing the food canal. Our large and small intestines have bacteria called E. coli, which are friendly in nature and help in digesting the food. Buckwheat is helpful to E. coli and thus improves the medium inside the large and small intestine. That helps to prevent irritable bowel syndrome and Crohn's disease, conditions that affect the colon adversely. It can effectively treat the issues related to constipation due to high concentrations of fiber.

Capers:

The importance of this root plant in traditional Chinese herbalism is well known. It is considered a great root to promote the self-healing capacity of the body and to maintain vital forces inside the body. Some western herbalists also used this root as the primary source of tonic, which is essential to promote natural immunity and vital capacities of the body. This root has some fantastic impacts on neural and endocrinal systems of the body. It can be a primary herbal remedy for patients with deficient immunity or those who are treated by chemotherapy and radiotherapy.

These benefits of the herb make it a herbal remedy of choice for cancer patients all over the world. It is a primary adaptive herbal remedy in oncology. Moreover, the use of astragalus is hazard-free and safe. It has a fantastic impact on bone marrow, and thus, it can easily promote immunity by producing more potent white blood cells that can be used in the war against the deadly pathogens like bacteria and viruses. It is very high in concentrations of polyphenols, which help in reducing body fats from the body.

Celery:

Much like to buckwheat, celery is very important for our stomach and intestine. Stomach acids, disturbed gut mobility, and injured food canal (esophagus) cause heartburn, a condition that affects every human many times in their lives. Celery prevents heartburn by improving the capacities of the stomach and colon as well as by healing the food canal. Our large and small intestines have bacteria called E. coli, which are friendly in nature and help in digesting the food. Buckwheat is helpful to E. coli and thus improves the medium inside the large and small intestine. That helps to prevent irritable bowel syndrome and Crohn's disease, conditions that affect the colon adversely. It can effectively treat the issues related to constipation due to high concentrations of fiber.

Chilies:

Chilis are used in both western and eastern foods and can be utilized to achieve higher metabolic rates because these are rich in capsicum. Capsicum is a potent fat mobilizer that can be used to break adipose tissues into much simpler precursors called fatty acid. Its action is dual. When these free fatty acids reach in our blood, the action of capsicum in chilies is to increase the basal metabolic rate, which is highly essential to burn these extra fatty acids in the bloodstream and thus promoting a lean physique without extra fat.

Cocoa:

Cocoa is very important for the brain. By improving overall health and through its antioxidant properties, cocoa can reduce the chances of dementia, Parkinsonism, and much other related pathology. Fatigue is another crucial aspect to be tackled here. Mental fatigue is related to the exhausting of the brain after prolonged functioning or reduced brain capacities, which can lead to general body pains and low self-esteem. By providing the nutritional supply to the brain, cocoa can help to prevent the mental as well as general fatigue.

Coffee:

Coffee is the reason for the popularity of the sirtfood diet. This diet regime allows the intake of caffeine in the body so that it can help in breaking the adipose tissues into fatty acid. Coffee, especially caffeine anhydrous, is beneficial in the mobilization of fats. Moreover, coffee also helps in reducing the fatigue in the brain, and it helps in the promotion of mental alertness. It is the biggest cause that the sirtfood diet provides mental focus and alertness to its users, which is not provided in many other ordinary fat loss diet plans.

extra virgin olive oil:

olive oil is the most used type of oil throughout the globe. Italian and French diets primarily include olive oils in the main course. Extra virgin olive oil is the lightest form of olive oil. It provides many polyunsaturated fatty acids, which are actually high-density lipids. These fatty acids are essential in the reduction of blood cholesterol levels as well as they are a vital energy source in the body. Olive oil is well-researched about its benefits on the brain and cardiac health, and honestly, this attempt is not sufficient to describe the benefits of olive oil.

Green tea:

Green tea is one of the most used types of tea around the world because of its health benefits. Green tea is well-researched about its benefits on the brain and cardiac health, and honestly, this writing is not sufficient to describe the benefits of olive oil. Green tea has rich historical importance in Indian ayurvedic medicine as well as in traditional western medicine. It was widely used to promote attention, focus, long-term and short-term memory, and brainpower in both children and adults. It was also used as an effective tonic for the heart and vascular health. In some literature, it is also shown that it was also used in lung diseases.

Red wine:

The first evidence of grapes was found in Egyptian culture, and they were cultivated at the bank of Neil River. The literature is not complete to build a consensus that grapes were used in Egyptian civilization, but it is clear that they were very fond of wine even they were the first one who introduced it. So, it can be possible that they did enjoy the taste of red grape wine. However, history shows that once the drink was introduced, it spread at a swift pace over different zones of the globe, much like we are observing it today. In 55 B.C. after the arrival of Roman in British waters, they found locals enjoying a traditional cider-like drink, which appealed to them too, and soon, it was being considered as one of their favorite beverages. So, this beverage, with small changes in the recipe, was introduced in the Roman Empire and then to Europe. It was the most popular drink of Germanic heritage, and they added it to the Normans. When Normans defeated the British Empire in the 9th century, they brought the word "wine" into the English dictionary.

In many other fat loss diets, wine is a prohibited drink, but the sirtfood diet is unique in this regard. The sirtfood diet allows the use of red grape wine, and even it is an essential part of the sirtfood diet because of many health benefits assured by red grape wine.

Other foods which mark the top twenty list of the sirtfood diet are:

Garlic

Kale

Medjool dates

Parsley

Red endive

Red onion

Soy

Strawberries

Turmeric

Walnuts

The green juice:

An essential component of the sirtfood diet is a green juice, which is a signature to this diet plan. To make a green juice of the sirtfood diet, you will need two kale, some parsley with celery (with leaves) and green apple. Lemon juice is an essential part of the signature green fruit and adding green tea to it is a beautiful idea.

If you know the benefits of these fresh foods, you can imagine how strong it can be against extra fats in your body. It is also very essential for your gut. Stomach acids, disturbed gut mobility, and injured food canal (esophagus) cause heartburn, a condition that affects every human many times in their lives. This juice prevents heartburn by improving the capacities of the stomach and colon as well as by healing the food canal. Our large and small intestines have bacteria called E. coli, which are friendly in nature and help in digesting the food. Buckwheat is helpful to E. coli and thus improves the medium inside the large and small intestine. That helps to prevent irritable bowel syndrome and Crohn's disease, conditions that affect the colon adversely. It can effectively treat the issues related to constipation due to high concentrations of fiber.

During the first three days of week one, you should drink three glass of this green juice daily. In the coming four days of week one, two glass of green juice is essential. Then in the second week, one glass per day is sufficient to unlock the health benefits.

Chapter 4: The Stages Of The Sirtfood Diet

Eating some quality foods will improve your "skinny gene" pathways and enables you to shed some unnecessary weight in seven days. Food such as kale, dark chocolate, and wine has a natural compound known as polyphenols that look likes the results of fitness workout and fasting. Strawberries, cinnamon, as well as turmeric are also strong sirtfoods. These foods will activate the sirtuin steps or potential to help improve weight loss.

There are 2 phases to follow the sirtfood diet:

PHASE 1 OF THE SIRTFOOD DIET

All through the first 3 days, calorie consumption is reduced to 1,000 calories (that is more than on a 5:2 fasting day). The diet involves 3 Sirtfood-full of green juices and 1 Sirtfood filled meal and 2 serves of dark chocolate.

For the remaining 4 days calories intake has to be increased to 1.500 calories and daily day the diet should involves 2 Sirtfood-filled green juices and 2 Sirtfood-rich meals.

In the early first stage "The phase 1 stage" you are not permitted to drink any alcohol, but you are free to take water and green tea.

PHASE 2 OF THE SIRTFOOD DIET

Phase 2 does not center on calorie intake reduction. Daily intake involves 3 Sirtfood-rich foods and 1 green juice, and the alternative of 1 or 2 Sirtfood crunch snacks, if necessary.

In the second phase 2 you are permitted to take red wine, but not too much (they advise you to take 2-3 glasses of red wine weekly), and also water, tea, coffee and green tea.

After the Diet

You may replicate these two phases as much you desired for additional weight loss.

However, you are advised to continue "sirtifying" your diet at the end of completing these phases by including sirtfoods frequently into your meals.

There are a variations of Sirtfood Diet manuals that has several recipes rich in sirtfoods. You can also add sirtfoods in your foods as a snack or in recipes you have used. In addition, you are advised to continue taking the green juice daily.

In this manner, the Sirtfood Diet will be more of a way of lifestyle adjustment than a one-time diet.

Diet to activate sirtuins and promote health

It's apparently no accident that some of the individuals with long lifespan and healthiest populations in the world eat diets that are rich in these sirtuin activating foods, examples are those in the Mediterranean and parts of Asia. The Mediterranean diet includes polyphenol rich fruits, veggies, olive oil including red wine. The Asian diet is rich in isoflavones present in soya beans and epigallactins from green tea.

Acquiring several of these health developing foods into your diet is proportionately easy. They can be included into many diets and even compound to make super-sirt meals!

Below are some grate ideas you can get started with

- Make use olive oil for frying or roasting veggies or vegetables and salad dressings.

- Ensure to own a jar of olives handy to snack on and include olives to salads or cooked meals. Tapenade usually makes a great topping for rye breads.

- Exchange usual tea and coffee for green tea. Include a press of lemon for extra interest.

- Miso alternatively can be used rather than stock cubes to flavor soups and stews. Milder light-colored miso may be used as a spread. Miso soup makes a great snack or soft meal if presented with salad or bread.

- Include tofu or tempeh to stir fries. Mix silken tofu into soups, immerse and creamy desserts.

- Buckwheat macaroni can be made as a tasty gluten complimentary option to wheat pasta and buckwheat flour can be made also in baked products or to stiffer sauces. Buckwheat is also a great alternative that goes well with salads combined with roasted vegetables and toasted nuts.

Chapter 5. What The Experts Think And Why You Lose Weight

The writers of the Sirtfood Diet say it's a way to move weight without significantly dieting as it stimulates the same receptors of the 'skinny gene' normally caused by fasting and exercise. "These foods contain chemicals called polyphenols that exert mild stress on our cells, leading to genes that mimic the fasting and exercise results. Foods rich in polyphenols these as broccoli, dark chocolate, and red wine activate sirtuin receptors that affect appetite, aging, and mood.

Research promoting the notion of foods like chili and green tea for weight loss and red wine (rich in polyphenols) is frequently quoted in the French paradox, which is why French people drink red wine but stay slim. However, there is no scientific proof to date that we can rely on that the sirtfood hypothesis is working.

The Sirtfood diet was known as the "alternative to traditional diets," according to Goggins. He and his partner, Glen Matten, were both "nutrition skeptics," because of their experience as natural health experts. The Sirtfood diet focuses on activating the sirtuin genes instead of focusing on weight reduction.

"The decrease of weight is not the primary objective, but as part of the biochemical rejuvenation of our cell well-being, which slowly resets our metabolism," Goggins said. "In comparison, unlike certain conventional diets that focus on cutting goods, we can only enjoy the advantages of consuming Sirtfoods, which means indulging in your favorite foods and not limiting them."

Kirkpatrick, who works with Cleveland Clinic in Ohio, said she had patients coming several times to ask her about the Sirtfood diet. While there is some evidence to support its results, she said all of the research and observations are very new.

"I think the diet is healthy because we don't have any evidence to show it's longevity in the long run," she said. "The entire premise behind the diet is that certain foods will induce certain sirtuins which are related to the body's proteins."

Kirkpatrick noted that the Sirtfood diet works in the same way as intermittent fasting diets which were also shown to help with weight loss.

Goggins said they were "increasingly obsessed" with "increasingly unhealthy eating habits" and people were "villainizing" products while he and Matten trained at the high-end private fitness club in London.

"Sugar will terrify you," he said. "And all of that was about calorie consumption cuts."

They needed to ensure that people were able to consume more of their preferred foods to have essential nutrients as they shaped their diet.

"It's important that we not only have enough of these foods in our diet but also make sure that our meals contain a number of them because they're the mixture of their meal and juice from which the real benefits come," Googins said.

A nutritionist 's final thoughts on the Sirtfood Diet

Michele says it's no surprise people will see a rapid weight loss if they reduce their calorie intake, especially during the first week of the diet. Still, she says she's very careful about encouraging people to count calories.

Nonetheless, she sees a big advantage in growing your dietary intake based on sirtuin, saying that any diet high in whole foods without adding sugars will improve your Health.

"Sirtfoods induce fat burning but also facilitate muscle growth, regeneration, and repair. Eating foods that are naturally abundant in sirtuin activators as an alternative to polyphenol supplements could be healthier, more efficient – and cheaper, "she added.

Yeah, you got it. While the Sirtfood diet has the right idea to promote the rise in whole food we can eat, the calorie counting motivation isn't exactly the healthiest path you might take on your well-being journey.

This is also a huge step towards a healthy, more appropriate lifestyle to focus on keeping a balanced, sirt-rich diet and adding physical fitness into the daytime.

Chapter 6: Sirtuins: Super Metabolic Regulators

What makes the Sirtfood Diet so strong is their ability to turn to an ancient gene family that exists within each of us. The name for that gene family is sirtuin. Sirtuins are unique in that they orchestrate processes deep within our cells that affect things as important as our ability to burn fat, our vulnerability to disease — or not — and ultimately even our life span. The influence of sirtuins is so deep that they are now called "the chief metabolic regulators." Basically, what exactly someone who wants to lose a few pounds and live a long and happy life will want to be in control.

In recent years, sirtuins have, unsurprisingly, become the subject of intense scientific research. The first sirtuin was discovered in yeast back in 1984, and research really began in the course of the coming three decades when it was revealed that sirtuin activation increases life span, first in yeast, and then all the way up to mice.

Why the thrills? Because the basic principles of cellular metabolism are almost identical from yeast to humans and everything in between. If you can manipulate something as tiny as budding yeast and see a benefit, then repeat it in higher organisms like mice, there is potential for the same benefits to be realized in humans.

That takes us to fast. Consistently, the lifelong limitation of food consumption has been shown to increase the life span of lower species and mammals. This remarkable finding is the basis for the practice of calories restriction for some people, where daily calorie consumption is decreased by 10 percent, as well as its popularized offshoot, intermittent fasting, which has become a common weight-loss diet, made famous by the likes of the 5:2

diet, or Fast Diet. Although we are still awaiting evidence of improved longevity for humans from these activities, there is evidence of benefits to what we could call "healthspan "— chronic diseases are declining, and fat is starting to melt away.

But let's be honest, no matter how significant the advantages, fasting week in, week out, is a grueling business that most of us don't want to sign up for. Even if we do, most of us are not willing to stick to this. Besides this, there are disadvantages to fasting, especially if we follow it for a long time. We listed in the introduction the side effects of hunger, irritability, fatigue, muscle loss, and slowing in metabolism. However, ongoing fasting schemes may also put us at risk of malnutrition, impacting our well-being due to a decreased intake of vital nutrients. Fasting schemes are often entirely inadequate for significant proportions of the population, such as infants, pregnant women, and most likely older adults. Although fasting has clearly proven benefits, it's not the magic bullet we'd like it to be. This makes us ask, is this really the way nature was supposed to make us slim and healthy? There's definitely a safer way out there.

Our breakthrough came when we discovered that the profound benefits of calorie restriction and fasting were mediated by triggering our ancient sirtuin genes 5. To better understand this, it might be beneficial to think of sirtuins as the guardians at the crossroads of energy status and longevity. Therefore, what they do is to respond to stress in the body.

When energy is in short supply, there is a rise in tension on our cells, just as we see in the caloric restriction. The sirtuins sensed this, and then turned on and transmitted a series of powerful signals that dramatically altered the behavior of cells. Sirtuins ramp up our metabolism, increase our muscle's efficiency, turn on fat burning, minimize inflammation, and repair any cell damage. Sirtuins, in turn, makes us fitter, leaner, and safer.

A Passion for Exercise?

It's not just caloric restriction and fasting that stimulates sirtuins; exercise also does. Sirtuins orchestrate the profound benefits of exercise much as in fasting. But while we are encouraged to participate in routine, moderate exercise for its multitude of benefits is recommended, it is not the means by which we are expected to focus our efforts on weight-loss. Research indicates that the human body has developed ways of adapting naturally and that the amount of energy that we use while exercising, which means that in order for exercise to be a successful weight-loss strategy, we need to devote considerable time and effort. That grueling workout regimen is the way nature intended us to maintain a healthy weight loss; this is even more questionable in the light of studies, now indicating that too much exercise can be harmful — weakening our immune systems, damaging the heart and leading to an early death.

Enter Sirtfoods

So far, we have discovered that triggering our sirtuin genes is vital if we want to lose weight and be healthy. Fasting and exercise have been the two known ways of doing this up till now. Unfortunately, the amounts needed for successful weight loss come with their drawbacks, and for most of us, it's merely incompatible with how we live twenty-first century lives. Luckily, there is a newly discovered, ground-breaking way to activate our sirtuin genes in the best way possible: sirtfood. As we'll soon know, these are the wonder foods that are particularly rich in specific natural plant chemicals that have the power to talk to our sirtuin genes and turn them on. In turn, they mimic the results of fasting and exercise and, in doing so, offer impressive benefits of burning fat, muscle building, and health-boosting that were once unachievable.

DEALING WITH THE FAT

One of the dramatic results from our Sirtfood Diet pilot study was not just the amount of weight the participants lost, which was very impressive — it was the sort of weight loss that really excited us. What caught our attention was the fact that a lot of people lost weight without losing any muscle. In reality, seeing people grow muscle wasn't uncommon. This left us with an inevitable conclusion: fat had merely melted away.

Achieving a significant fat loss normally requires a considerable sacrifice, either severely reducing calories or engaging in superhuman exercise levels or both. Contrary to that, our participants either maintained or lowered their level of exercise and did not even report feeling particularly hungry. In reality, some even struggled to eat all of the food they had been provided with.

How is it even possible? Only when we understand what happens to our fat cells when there is an increased sirtuin activity, then we begin to make sense of these incredible findings.

LEAN GENES

Mice genetically engineered with high levels of SIRT1, the sirtuin gene that causes fat loss, are leaner and more metabolically active, 1 whereas mice without SIRT1 are fatter and have more metabolic disease. 2 When we look at humans, levels of SIRT1 have been found to be significantly lower in obese people's body fat than their healthy weight counts. This is because we get benefits on several levels by sirtuins, beginning at the very root of everything: the genes that regulate weight gain.

To understand this further, we need to look deeper into what is happening in our bodies, which is causing us to gain some weight.

FAT BUSTING

We will explain this in terms of a drug-ring in Hollywood. The streets flooding with drugs is our body flooding with fat. The drug pushers on the street corners are the source of the weight gain peddling reactions in our bodies. But in fact, it's just the low-level thugs. The true villain is behind it all, masterminding the entire operation, directing every deal that the peddlers make. This antagonist is referred to in our film as PPAR-π (peroxisome proliferator-activated receptor-ÿ). PPAR-ÿ orchestrates the cycle of fat accumulation by switching on the genes needed to start synthesizing and storing fat.6 To avoid fat proliferation, you need to cut supply. Stop PPAR-ÿ, and you avoid fat benefit effectively.

Enter our hero SIRT1, who rises to bring the villain down. With the villain locked up tightly, there is no one to pull the trigger and the whole fat-gain enterprise crumbles. With PPAR-π's operation halted, SIRT1 is turning its focus to "cleaning the streets." Not only is this achieved by shutting down fat production and storage, as we have shown, but it is also altering our metabolism so that we begin to clear the body of excess fat. Like any good crime-fighting hero, SIRT1 has a sidekick, a central regulator known as PGC-1α in our cells. This effectively stimulates the formation of what is known as mitochondria. These are the tiny factories of energy that exist within each of our cells — the power the body. The more we have the mitochondria, the more we can generate the electricity. But as well as encouraging more mitochondria, PGC-1α also encourages them to burn fat as the fuel of choice to make the energy. Thus, fat accumulation is blocked on the one side, and fat burning on the other increases.

Chapter 7: Meal Planning In Relation To The Phases

The great flexibility of the Sirt diet, which according to scholars is divided into two phases, allows those who decide to follow it not to be strict in doing so, i.e. the two phases of which it is characterized can be repeated even only from time to time, according to our needs.

Step 1 - Slimming

Phase 1 is also known as slimming time and lasts seven days. This is the hardest phase because you take fewer calories and the diet is less varied. The first 2-3 days should not exceed 1000 kcal so that the diet will consist of three green or centrifuged juices accompanied by a single solid meal. From the third day on, calories can increase to 1500 kcal, eating two green (or centrifuged) juices together with two solid meals.

It is the "supersonic" phase precisely because this week the slimming is well evident.

Phase 2 – Maintenance

Phase 2 lasts about two weeks and is used to preserve and maintain the weight loss.

Nutritionists recommend three solid meals to choose from the Sirt foods already mentioned + a green maintenance juice. The calories not to be exceeded reach 2,000 kcal, but at this stage, more outbursts are allowed with glasses of wine and vegetables at will.

HOW IT WORKS (how to lose 3.5 lbs. in just 7 days)

The first 7 days are the most difficult, as you can consume a maximum of 1000 calories per day in the first 3 days, then 1500 calories from day 3 to day 7. The menus are based on smoothies and centrifuged vegetables (the so-called green juices) in the first 3 days, with only one solid meal of your choice, but always based on Sirt food cooked with ad-hoc preparation (a light preparation may still be fine). From day four, with an additional 500 calories you can add an additional solid meal. In the first week, the Diet Sirt allows you to lose just over 3 kg.

The second phase goes from the 8th to the 21st day and includes three solid meals a day, plenty of Sirt food (but I remain in a range of 2000kcal) and a green juice based on Sirt vegetables.

Here is the preparation of centrifuged green juice. The green juice has the ability to purify and satiate and will be the protagonist of the first week of food plan.

To prepare it, it takes:

- 75 g kale
- 30 g arugula
- 5 g parsley
- 150 g green celery with leaves
- 1/2 green apple
- 1/2 lemon juice
- 1/2 teaspoon satin matcha teaspoon

Preparation Centrifuge

The kale, rocket and parsley; add celery and grated apple; enrich with half a squeezed lemon and half teaspoon of matcha tea. Drink immediately so as not to lose the beneficial effects of vegetables and not to store it in the fridge. It must always be prepared at the time of consumption.

The green juice should be consumed half an hour before breakfast, lunch and dinner and possibly never eat more than 7 p.m..

Chapter 8: Breakfast

1 Sirtfood Breakfast Scramble

Preparation Time: 10 minutes

Cooking Time: 10 minutes

Servings: 2

Ingredients:

1 tsp mild curry powder

½ bird's eye chili, thinly sliced

Two eggs

1 tsp ground turmeric

A handful of button mushrooms, thinly sliced

5g parsley, finely chopped

20g kale, roughly chopped

1 tsp extra virgin olive oil

Directions:

Combine the curry and turmeric powder, then apply a little water until a soft paste has been produced.

Steam up the kale 2–3 minutes.

You have to heat the oil over medium flame in a frying pan and fry the chili and mushrooms for 2–3 minutes before they start browning and softening.

Insert the eggs and spice paste, then cook over medium heat, then insert the kale and continue cooking for another minute over medium heat. Add the parsley, then blend well and serve.

Nutrition:

Calories: 174 Cal

Fat: 12.16 g

Protein: 10.57 g

Sugar: 1.3 g

2 Summer Berry Smoothie

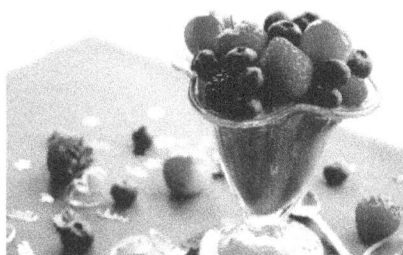

Preparation Time: 10 minutes

Cooking Time: 10 minutes

Servings: 1-2

Ingredients:

1 1/2 cups frozen mixed berries

3/4 cup vanilla Greek yogurt

One tablespoon honey optional

1 1/2 cups apple juice (you can also use skim milk, almond milk, coconut milk or other flavors of juice)

One banana sliced

Fresh berries and mint sprigs (optional step if you want to garnish)

Directions:

In a blender, put the apple juice, banana, berries, and yogurt; blend until smooth. If the smoothie seems too dense, add the liquid (1/4 cup) a bit more.

Taste and, if necessary, incorporate the sugar. You can garnish with fresh berries and mint sprigs if needed, then serve into two cups.

Nutrition:

Calories: 221 Cal

Fat: 1 g

Protein: 24 g

Sugar: 41 g

3 Rocket And Arugula Salad

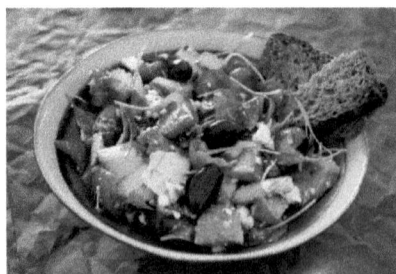

Preparation Time: 10 minutes

Cooking Time: 10 minutes

Servings: 2 -3

Ingredients:

40 gm rocket leaves

30 ml red wine

Salt as required

1 cup arugula

80 gm pear

10 gm toasted walnuts

10 gm yogurt (curd)

Powdered black pepper as required

Dressing:

13 ml virgin olive oil

30 ml of lemon juice

30 ml balsamic vinegar

Directions:

Wash the pears in running water, peel and cut them into thin slices. Soak them up and cool them in a small bowl of red wine.

Whisk balsamic vinegar, virgin olive oil, and lemon juice together in a cup to make the dressing for the salad. With this sauce, mix the rocket and arugula in a medium bowl and mix salt and black pepper powder over the leaves.

Put the poached pears nicely around the salad and top with yogurt and toasted walnuts.

Nutrition:

Calories: 322 Cal

Fat: 3.59 g

Protein: 5.56 g

Sugar: 36.7 g

4 Vegan Kale Salad With Cranberries

Preparation Time: 10 minutes

Cooking Time: 0 minutes

Servings: 2

Ingredients:

¼ cup dried cranberries

One dash salt optional

¼ cup pine nuts or other chopped nuts optional

6 cups of shredded kale

1/3 cup Maple Vinaigrette Dressing

Directions:

Wash well, kale.

Rip it into tiny bits by removing the rough stem.

Drizzle over the Maple Vinaigrette Dressing by putting in a big bowl.

Sprinkle with a bit of salt (optional)

Massage the dressing onto the kale with your palms until it becomes light green and shiny.

If wanted, sprinkle with dried cranberries and cover with almonds.

*Recipe notes:

You can enjoy this salad straight away or leave it in the fridge for a couple of hours before it's ready to serve.

This is safest if you feed within 12 hours of preparing this.

Nutrition:

Calories: 215 Cal

Fat: 2.12 g

Protein: 4.96 g

Sugar: 23.74 g

5 Mushroom Buckwheat Pancakes

Preparation Time: 10 minutes

Cooking Time: 15 minutes

Servings: 3 - 5

Ingredients:

55g whole meal flour

55g buckwheat flour

275ml Alpro Almond Milk

One free-range egg

30g butter, for frying

For the filling:

50g flour

50g butter

100g sliced chestnut mushrooms

Three large handfuls of baby spinach

Olive oil

Directions:

Melt butter in a saucepan of 50 g. Insert the flour to form a paste. Start cooking for 30 seconds.

Gradually add the milk, stirring vigorously until the white sauce is smooth. (Make sure to mix properly so that lumps do not form.)

Fry the mushrooms in the oil until the spinach is brown and wilt. Drop the mushrooms into the white sauce, apply the cheese and nutmeg to taste, then season.

In the meanwhile, add the two flour forms to a pot, and create a little well.

Whisk the egg into the milk, lightly. Pour a few of the egg mixture into the flour and start whisking. Start inserting the liquid and whisking until the batter is smooth.

Melt the butter and apply a ladle of the batter in a non-stick frying pan. Swirl for coating the base of the pan evenly and flip it when the pancake becomes able to shake. Repeat until all the batter has been consumed, and then fill it with mushroom and spinach stuffing.

Nutrition:

Calories: 298 Cal

Fat: 77.6 g

Protein: 30.52 g

Sugar: 4.39 g

6 Chicory And Nut Salad

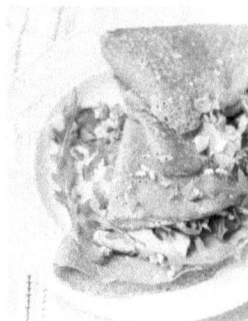

Preparation Time: 10 minutes

Cooking Time: 5 minutes

Servings 2 - 3

Ingredients:

1/2 teaspoon Dijon mustard

Salt and freshly ground black pepper

1/2-pound chicory, or other leafy green

1/4 cup shaved parmesan

1/2 cup coarsely chopped walnuts

1 tablespoon sherry vinegar

3 tablespoons walnut oil

Directions:

You have to toast the nuts in a dry skillet over medium-high heat until they are fragrant, around 2 minutes. Set aside to cool down.

Whisk the vinegar, oil, mustard, salt, and pepper together in a tiny cup, to taste.

Place the chicory in a wide bowl with the coating. Put walnuts on the serving plates and top, and rasp parmesan.

Nutrition:

Calories: 282 Cal

Fat: 68.2 g

Protein: 17.36 g

Sugar: 21.23 g

7 Honey, Garlic And Chili Oven-Roasted Squash
Preparation Time: 15 minutes

Cooking Time: 40 minutes

Servings: 3

Ingredients:

1 kg assorted squash and pumpkin (at least five different types), cut in medium size pieces

4 red or green chilies

Two sprigs thyme

3 Tbsp (15 ml) honey

 3 Tbsp (15 ml) olive oil

Three whole garlic cloves, lightly crushed

One sprig rosemary

Salt and pepper to taste

Directions:

Preheat your oven to 150 ° C.

Place all the supplements in a wide bowl and require standing for 30 minutes, stirring periodically.

In a roasting tray, put the squash and cover with foil.

Roast covered at 150 ° C for 10 minutes.

Increase the temperature of the oven to 180 ° C, remove the foil, and roast for another 10 minutes allowing the squash to caramelize lightly.

Nutrition:

Calories: 323 Cal

Fat: 162 g

Protein: 14 g

Sugar: 61 g

8 Sirtfood Mushroom Scramble Eggs

Preparation Time: 10 minutes

Cooking Time: 10 minutes

Servings: 4

Ingredients:

2 tbsp

1 teaspoon ground garlic

1 teaspoon mild curry powder

20g lettuce, approximately sliced

1 teaspoon extra virgin olive oil

1/2 bird's eye peeled, thinly chopped

a couple of mushrooms, finely chopped

5g parsley, finely chopped

*elective * Insert a seed mix for a topper plus Some Rooster Sauce for taste

Directions:

Mix the curry and garlic powder and then add just a little water till you've achieved a light glue.

Steam the lettuce for two -- 3 minutes.

Heat the oil in a skillet over a moderate heat and fry the chili and mushrooms 2-- three minutes till they've begun to soften and brown.

Insert the eggs and spice paste and cook over moderate heat, then add the carrot and then proceed to cook over a moderate heat for a further minute. In the end, put in the parsley, mix well, and function.

Nutrition:

Calories: 43 Cal

Fat: 2.33 g

Protein: 1.25 g

Sugar: 0.39 g

9 Turkey Breakfast Sausages

Preparation Time: 15 minutes

Cooking Time: 20 minutes

Servings: 2

Ingredients:

1 lb. extra lean ground turkey

1 Tbsp EVOO, and a little more to dirt pan

1 Tbsp fennel seeds

2 teaspoons smoked paprika

1 teaspoon red pepper flakes

1 teaspoon peppermint

1 teaspoon chicken seasoning

A couple of shredded cheddar cheese

A couple of chives, finely chopped

A few shakes garlic and onion powder

Two spins of pepper and salt

Directions:

Pre Heat oven to 350F.

Utilize a little EVOO to dirt a miniature muffin pan.

Combine all ingredients and blend thoroughly.

Fill each pit on top of the pan and then cook for approximately 15-20 minutes. Each toaster differs; therefore, when muffin fever is 165, then remove.

Nutrition:

Calories: 168 Cal

Fat: 44.71 g

Protein: 285.92 g

Sugar: 3.71 g

10banana And Blueberry Muffins - Src

Preparation Time: 20 minutes

Cooking Time: 30 minutes

Servings: 10

Ingredients:

4 large ripe bananas, peeled and mashed

3/4 cup of sugar

1 egg, lightly crushed

1/2 cup of butter, melted (and a little extra to dust the interiors of this muffin tin)

2 cups of blueberries (if they are suspended, do not Defrost them. simply pop them into the batter suspended)

1 teaspoon baking powder

1 teaspoon baking soda

1/2 teaspoon salt

1 cup of coconut bread

1/2 cup of flour (or 1-1; two cup bread)

1/2 cup applesauce

dab of cinnamon

Directions:

Add mashed banana to a large mixing bowl.

Insert sugar & egg and mix well.

Add peanut butter and strawberries.

Sift all the dry ingredients together, then add the dry ingredients into the wet mix and mix together lightly.

Set into 12 greased muffin cups

Bake for 20-30min in 180C or 350 F.

Nutrition:

Calories: 203 Cal

Fat: 106.48 g

Protein: 21.8 g

Sugar: 196 g

11easy Egg-White Muffins

Preparation Time: 20 minutes

Cooking Time: 1 hour

Servings: 8

Ingredients:

Language muffin - I enjoy Ezekiel 7 grain

egg-whites - 6 tbsp or two large egg whites

turkey bacon or bacon sausage

sharp cheddar cheese or gouda

green berry

discretionary - lettuce, and hot sauce, hummus, flaxseeds, etc.

Directions:

At a microwavable safe container, then spray entirely to stop the egg from adhering, then pour egg whites into the dish.

Lay turkey bacon or bacon sausage paper towel and then cook.

Subsequently, toast your muffin, if preferred.

Then put the egg dish in the microwave for 30 minutes. Afterward, with a spoon or fork, then immediately flip egg within the dish and cook for another 30 minutes.

Whilst dish remains hot sprinkle some cheese while preparing sausage.

The secret is to get a paste of some kind between each coating to put up the sandwich together, i.e., a very small little bit of hummus or even cheese.

Nutrition:

Calories: 837 Cal

Fat: 34.95 g

Protein: 14.71 g

Sugar: 68.61 g

12sweet Potato Hash

Preparation Time: 10 minutes

Cooking Time: 10 minutes

Servings: 4

Ingredients:

Inch Sweet potato

1/2 red pepper, diced

3 green onions, peppermint

leftover turkey, then sliced into bits (optional)

1 Tbsp of butter - perhaps a bit less (I never quantify)

carrot powder - a few shakes

Pepper - only a small dab to get a bit of warmth

pepper and salt to flavor

scatter of cheddar cheese (optional)

Directions:

Stab a sweet potato and microwave for 5 minutes.

Remove from microwave, peel the skin off, and foliage.

At a skillet, on medium-high warmth, place peppers and butter and sauté to get a few minutes.

Insert potato bits and keep sautéing.

Whilst sauté, add sweeteners, leafy vegetables, and green onions.

Insert a dab of cheddar and Revel in!

Nutrition:

Calories: 145 Cal

Fat: 11.79 g

Protein: 1.79 g

Sugar: 5.08 g

13asparagus, Mushroom Artichoke Strata

Preparation Time: 20 minutes

Cooking Time: 15 minutes

Servings: 2

Ingredients:

Inch little loaf of sourdough bread

4 challah rolls

8 eggs

2 cups of milk

1 teaspoon salt

1/4 teaspoon black pepper

1 cup Fontina cheese, cut into little chunks

1/2 cup shredded Parmesan cheese

1 Tbsp butter (I used jojoba)

1 teaspoon dried mustard

1/2 can of artichoke hearts, sliced

1 bunch green onions, grated

1 bunch asparagus, cut into 1-inch bits

1 10oz package of baby Bella (cremini) mushrooms, chopped

Directions:

Clean mushrooms and slice and trim asparagus and cut in 1-inch pieces. Reserve in a bowl and scatter 1/2 teaspoon salt mixture.

Drain and dice 1/2 may or modest artichoke hearts.

Melt butter in a pan over moderate heat, also sauté the asparagus and mushrooms before the mushrooms start to brown, about 10 minutes.

Blend the artichoke core pieces into a bowl with all a mushroom/asparagus mix. Set aside.

Cut or split a tiny sourdough loaf into 1-inch bits. (My loaf was a little too small, therefore that I used 4 challah rolls too)

Grease a 9x13 inch baking dish and generate a base coating of bread at the dish. Spread 1/2 cup of Fontina cheese bread, at a coating, and disperse half an apple mixture on the cheese.

Lay-down a different layer of these vegetables and bread and high using a 1/2 cup of Fontina cheese.

Whisk together eggs, salt, milk, dry mustard, and pepper into a bowl and then pour the egg mixture on the vegetables and bread.

Cover the dish, and then simmer for 3 weeks.

Pre Heat oven to 375 degrees.

Eliminate the casserole from the fridge and let stand for half an hour.

Spread All the Parmesan cheese at a coating within the strata.

Bake in the preheated oven until a time when a knife inserted near the border comes out clean, 40 to 45 minutes. Allow it stand 5 to 10 minutes before cutting into squares.

Nutrition:

Calories: 350 Cal

Fat: 169 g

Protein: 181 g

Sugar: 49.76 g

Chapter 9: Soups And Salads

14spicy Squash Soup

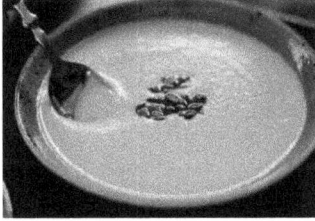

Preparation Time: 5 minutes

Cooking Time: 45 minutes

Servings: 4

Ingredients:

150g 5oz kale

1 butternut squash, peeled, de-seeded and chopped

1 red onion, chopped

3 bird's-eye chilies, chopped

3 cloves of garlic

2 teaspoons turmeric

1 teaspoon ground ginger

600 ml 1-pint vegetable stock broth

2 tablespoons olive oil

128 calories per serving

Directions:

Heat the olive oil in a saucepan, add the chopped butternut squash and onion and cook for 6 minutes until softened. Stir in the kale, garlic, chili, turmeric and ginger and cook for 2 minutes, stirring constantly. Pour in the vegetable stock broth bring it to the boil and cook for 20 minutes. Using a food processor or a hand blender process until smooth. Serve on its own or with a swirl of cream or crème fraiche. Enjoy.

Nutrition:

Calories: 258 Cal

Fat: 28.82 g

Protein: 8.94 g

Sugar: 30.3 g

15butternut Pumpkin With Buckwheat

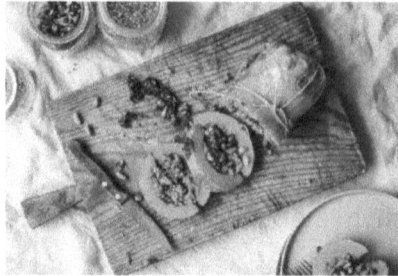

Preparation Time: 10 minutes

Cooking Time: 30 minutes

Servings: 4

Ingredients:

1 tablespoon of extra virgin olive oil

1 red onion, finely chopped

1 tablespoon fresh ginger, finely chopped

3 cloves of garlic, finely chopped

2 small chilies, finely chopped

1 tablespoon cumin

1 cinnamon stick

2 tablespoons turmeric

800g chopped canned tomatoes

300ml vegetable broth

100g dates, seeded and chopped

one 400g tin of chickpeas, drained

500g butter squash, peeled, seeded and cut into pieces

200g buckwheat

5g coriander, chopped

10g parsley, chopped

Directions:

Preheat oven to 400 °.

Heat the olive oil in a frying pan and sauté the onion, ginger, garlic and tai chili. After two minutes add cumin, cinnamon and turmeric and cook for another two minutes while stirring.

Add the tomatoes, dates, stock and chickpeas, stir well and cook over a low heat for 45 to 60 minutes. Add some water as required. In the meantime, mix the pumpkin pieces with olive oil and bake in the oven for about 30 minutes until soft.

Cook the buckwheat according to the Directions and add the remaining turmeric. When everything is cooked, add the pumpkin to the other ingredients in the roaster and serve with the buckwheat. Sprinkle with coriander and parsley.

Nutrition:

Calories: 298 Cal

Fat: 11 g

Protein: 24 g

Sugar: 6 g

16celery & Blue Cheese Soup

Preparation Time: 5 minutes

Cooking Time: 55 minutes

Servings: 4

Ingredients:

125g 4ozblue cheese

25g 1ozbutter

1 head of celery approx. 650g

1 red onion, chopped

900 ml 1½ pints chicken stock broth

150 ml 5fl oz single cream

Directions:

Heat the butter in a saucepan, add the onion and celery and cook until the vegetables have softened. Pour in the stock, bring to the boil then reduce the heat and simmer for 15 minutes. Pour in the cream and stir in the cheese until it has melted. Serve and eat straight away.

Nutrition:

Calories: 312 Cal

Fat: 92 g

Protein: 34 g

Sugar: 62.3 g

17cauliflower & Walnut Soup

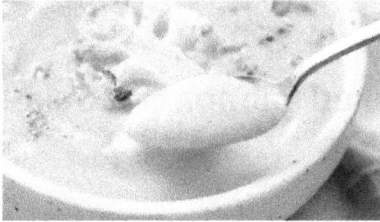

Preparation Time: 5 minutes

Cooking Time: 45 minutes

Servings:4

Ingredients:

450g 1lbcauliflower, chopped 8 walnut halves, chopped

1 red onion, chopped

900 ml 1½ pints vegetable stock broth

100mls 3½ fl. oz double cream heavy cream

½ teaspoon turmeric

1 tablespoon olive oil

249 calories per serving

Directions:

Heat the oil in a saucepan, add the cauliflower and red onion and cook for 4 minutes, stirring continuously. Pour in the stock broth), bring to the boil and cook for 15 minutes. Stir in the walnuts, double cream and turmeric. Using a food processor or hand blender, process the soup until smooth and creamy. Serve into bowls and top off with a sprinkling of chopped walnuts.

Nutrition:

Calories: 298 Cal

Fat: 11 g

Protein: 24 g

Sugar: 6 g

18smoked Salmon Sirt Salad

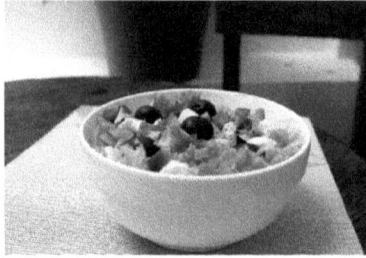

Preparation Time: 10 minutes

Cooking Time: 40 minutes

Servings: 4

Ingredients:

1 cup, or ¼ package if large of smoked salmon slices no cooking needed!

1 avocado, pitted, sliced, and scooped out

10 walnuts, chopped

5 lovage or celery leaves), chopped

2 celery stalks, chopped or sliced thinly

½ small red onion, sliced thinly

1 Medjool pitted date, chopped

1 tbsp. capers

1 tbsp. extra virgin olive oil

1/4 of a lemon, juiced

5 sprigs of parsley, chopped

Directions:

Wash and dry salad makings and vegetables, top with salmon.

Nutrition:

Calories: 238 Cal

Fat: 79.9 g

Protein: 187 g

Sugar: 56.9 g

19sirtfood Granola

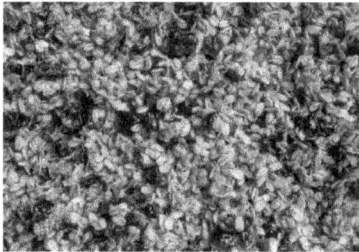

Preparation Time: 5 minutes

Cooking Time: 25 minutes

Servings: 4

Ingredients:

200g oats

250g buckwheat flakes

100g walnuts, chopped

100g almonds, chopped

100g dried strawberries

1 ½ tsp ground ginger

1 ½ tsp ground cinnamon

120mls olive oil

2 tbsp honey

Directions:

Preheat oven to 150C or gas mark 3. Line a tray with baking parchment.

Stir together walnuts, almonds, buckwheat flakes and oats with ginger and cinnamon. In a large pan, warm olive oil and honey, heating until the honey has dissolved.

Pour the honey-oil over the other ingredients, stirring to ensuring an even coating. Separate the granola evenly over the lined baking tray and roast for 50 minutes, or until golden.

Remove from the oven and leave to cool. Once cooled add the berries and store in an airtight container. Eat dry or with milk and yogurt. It stays fresh for up to 1 week.

Nutrition:

Calories: 213 Cal

Fat: 13.1 g

Protein: 80.62 g

Sugar: 51.67 g

20 tofu & Shiitake Mushroom Soup

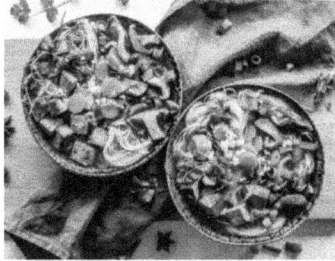

Preparation Time: 10 minutes

Cooking Time: 35 minutes

Servings: 4

Ingredients:

10g dried wakame

1L vegetable stock

200g shiitake mushrooms, sliced

120g miso paste

1* 400g firm tofu, diced

2 green onion, trimmed and diagonally chopped

1 bird's eye chili, finely chopped

Directions:

Soak the wakame in lukewarm water for 10-15 minutes before draining.

In a medium-sized saucepan add the vegetable stock and bring to the boil. Toss in the mushrooms and simmer for 2-3 minutes.

Mix miso paste with 3-4 tbsp of vegetable stock from the saucepan, until the miso is entirely dissolved. Pour the miso-stock back into the pan and add the tofu, wakame, green onions and chili, then serve immediately.

Nutrition:

Calories: 298 Cal

Fat: 11 g

Protein: 24 g

Sugar: 6 g

21chocolate Chips Granola

Preparation Time: 5 minutes

Cooking Time: 65 minutes

Servings: 8

Ingredients:

2 tablespoons of rice malt syrup

20g of butter

200g of jumbo oats

60g of good quality 70% dark chocolate chips

3 tablespoons of light olive oil 1 tablespoon of dark brown sugar

50g of roughly chopped pecans

Directions:

Preheat your oven to 160°C. Use baking parchment or silicone sheet to line a large baking tray.

Add the pecans and oats into a large bowl and mix.

Add butter, olive oil, rice malt syrup, and brown sugar to a small pan and gently heat until the butter melts and the syrup and sugar dissolves do not allow to boil).

Drizzle the syrup over the oats and stir thoroughly until the oats are fully coated. Distribute granola all over the baking tray and leave clumps of with a bit of spacing instead of an even spread. Allow to bake in the oven until you see a tinge of golden brown on the edges about 20 minutes).

Remove them and allow to cool. Once cooled, break up the bigger lumps and mix in chocolate chips. Serve and enjoy. Scoop the remaining granola into an airtight jar. It will keep for about 2 weeks.

Nutrition:

Calories: 298 Cal

Fat: 11 g

Protein: 24 g

Sugar: 6 g

22honey Chili Nuts

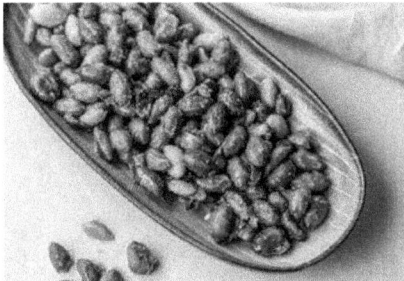

Preparation Time: 10 minutes

Cooking Time: 30 minutes

Servings: 4

Ingredients:

150g 5oz walnuts

150g 5oz pecan nuts

50g 2oz softened butter

1 tablespoon honey

½ bird's-eye chili, very finely chopped and de-seeded

126 calories per serving

Directions:

Preheat the oven to 180C/360F. Combine the butter, honey and chili in a bowl then add the nuts and stir them well. Spread the nuts onto a lined baking sheet and roast them in the oven for 10 minutes, stirring once halfway through. Remove from the oven and allow them to cool before eating.

Nutrition:

Calories: 428 Cal

Fat: 21 g

Protein: 37.7 g

Sugar: 61 g

23pomegranate Guacamole

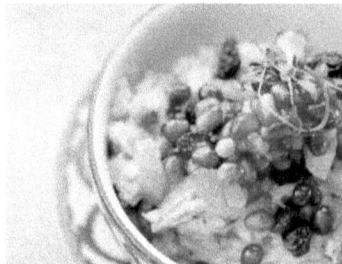

Preparation Time: 10 minutes

Cooking Time: 40 minutes

Servings: 4

Ingredients:

Flesh of 2 ripe avocados

Seeds from 1 pomegranate

1 bird's-eye chili pepper, finely chopped

½ red onion, finely chopped

Juice of 1 lime

151 calories per serving

Directions:

Place the avocado, onion, chill and lime juice into a blender and process until smooth. Stir in the pomegranate seeds. Chill before serving. Serve as a dip for chop vegetables.

Nutrition:

Calories: 298 Cal

Fat: 58.68 g

Protein: 8.22 g

Sugar: 36.6 g

Chapter 10: Lunch

24sticky Chicken Watermelon Noodle Salad

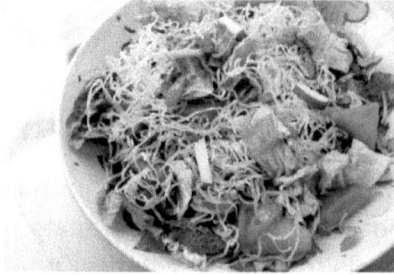

Preparation Time: 8 minutes

Cooking Time: 0 minutes

Servings: 3

Ingredients:

2 pieces of skinny rice noodles

1/2 Tbsp sesame oil

2 cups Watermelon

Head of bib lettuce

Half of a Lot of scallions

Half of a Lot of fresh cilantro

2 skinless, boneless chicken breasts

1/2 Tbsp Chinese five-spice

1 Tbsp extra virgin olive oil

two Tbsp sweet skillet (I utilized a mixture of maple syrup using a dash of Tabasco)

1 Tbsp sesame seeds

a couple of cashews - smashed

Dressing - could be made daily or 2 until

1 Tbsp low-salt soy sauce

1 teaspoon sesame oil

1 Tbsp peanut butter

Half of a refreshing red chili

Half of a couple of chives

Half of a couple of cilantros

1 lime - juiced

1 small spoonful of garlic

Directions:

At a bowl, then completely substituting the noodles in boiling drinking water. They are going to be soon carried out in 2 minutes.

On a big sheet of parchment paper, then throw the chicken with pepper, salt, and also the five-spice.

Twist over the newspaper, subsequently celebration and put the chicken using a rolling pin.

Place into the large skillet with 1 Tbsp of olive oil, turning 3 or 4 minutes, until well charred and cooked through.

Drain the noodles and toss with 1 Tbsp of sesame oil onto a sizable serving dish.

Place 50% the noodles into the moderate skillet, stirring frequently until crispy and nice.

Eliminate the Watermelon skin, then slice the flesh to inconsistent balls and then increase the platter.

Reduce the lettuces and cut into small wedges and also half of a whole lot of leafy greens and scatter the dish.

Place another 1 / 2 the cilantro pack, the soy sauce, coriander, chives, peanut butter, and a dab of water, 1 teaspoon of sesame oil and the lime juice, then mix till smooth.

Set the chicken back to heat, garnish with all the sweet skillet (or my walnut syrup mixture), and toss with the sesame seeds.

Pour the dressing on the salad toss gently with fresh fingers until well coated, then add crispy noodles and then smashed cashews.

Blend chicken pieces and add them to the salad.

Nutrition:

Calories: 555 Cal

Fat: 26.97 g

Protein: 14.55 g

Sugar: 53.16 g

25fruity Curry Chicken Salad

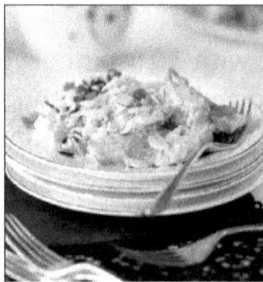

Preparation Time: 10 minutes

Cooking Time: 0 minutes

Servings: 1

Ingredients:

4 skinless, boneless Chicken Pliers - cooked and diced

1 tsp celery, diced

4 green onions, sliced

1 Golden Delicious apple peeled, cored and diced

1/3 cup golden raisins

1/3 cup seedless green grapes, halved

1/2 cup sliced toasted pecans

⅛ teaspoon ground black pepper

1/2 tsp curry powder

3/4 cup light mayonnaise

Directions:

In a big bowl, combine the chicken, onion, celery, apple, celery, celery, pecans, pepper, curry powder, and carrot. Mix altogether. Drink!

Nutrition:

Calories: 228 Cal

Fat: 93.59 g

Protein: 18.21 g

Sugar: 60.79 g

26lamb, Butternut Squash And Date Tagine

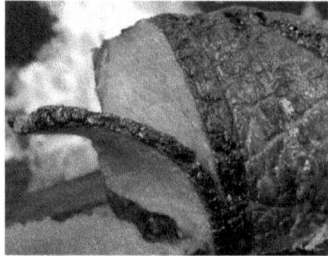

Incredible Warming Moroccan spices create this balanced tagine perfect for cold autumn and chilly evenings. Drink buckwheat to get an excess overall health kick!

Preparation Time: 15 minutes

Cooking Time: 20 minutes

Servings: 2 -3

Ingredients:

2 Tsp coconut oil

1 Red onion, chopped

2cm ginger, grated

3 Garlic cloves, crushed or grated

1 teaspoon chili flakes (or to taste)

2 Tsp cumin seeds

1 cinnamon stick

2 teaspoons ground turmeric

800g lamb neck fillet, cut into 2cm chunks

1/2 Tsp salt

100g Medjool dates, pitted and sliced

400g Tin chopped berries, and half of a can of plain water

500g Butternut squash, chopped into 1cm cubes

400g Tin chickpeas, drained

2 Tsp fresh coriander (and extra for garnish)

Buckwheat, Cous-cous, flatbread or rice to function

Directions:

Pre Heat Your oven to 140C.

Drizzle Roughly 2 tbsp of coconut oil into a large ovenproof saucepan or cast-iron casserole dish. Add the chopped onion and cook on a gentle heat, with the lid for around five minutes, until the onions are softened but not too brown.

Insert The grated ginger and garlic, chili, cumin, cinnamon, and garlic. Stir well and cook 1 minute with off the lid. Add a dash of water when it becomes too humid.

Then, add from the lamb balls. Stir to coat the beef from the spices and onions, then add the salt chopped meats and berries and roughly half of a can of plain water (100-200ml).

Bring The tagine into the boil and put the lid and put on your skillet for about 1 hour and fifteen minutes.

Ten Moments prior to the conclusion of this cooking period, add the chopped butternut squash and drained chickpeas. Stir everything together, place the lid back and go back to the oven to the last half an hour of cooking.

When That, the tagine is able to remove from the oven and then stir fry throughout the chopped coriander. Drink buckwheat, couscous, flatbread, or basmati rice.

Notes

In case You really do not have an ovenproof saucepan or cast-iron casserole dish, then only cook the tagine at a standard saucepan until it must go from the oven and transfer the tagine to a routine lidded skillet before placing in the oven. Add in an additional five minutes of cooking time and energy to allow the simple fact that the noodle dish will probably be needing additional time to warm up.

Nutrition:

Calories: 260 Cal

Fat: 111 g

Protein: 44 g

Sugar: 25.2 g

27turmeric Baked Salmon-Sirtfood Recipes

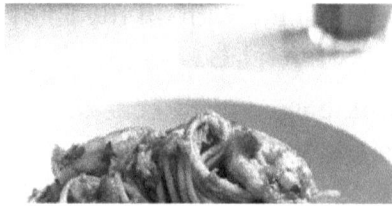

Preparation Time: 15 minutes

Cooking Time: 20 minutes

Servings: 3

Ingredients:

125-150 Gram Skinned Salmon

1 Tsp extra-virgin coconut oil

1 Tsp Ground turmeric

1/4 Juice of a lemon

To get The hot celery

1 Tsp extra-virgin coconut oil

40 G Red onion, finely chopped

60 Gram Tinned green peas

1 Garlic clove, finely chopped

1 Cm fresh ginger, finely chopped

1 Bird's eye chili, finely chopped

150 Gram Celery, cut into 2cm lengths

1 Tsp darkened curry powder

130 Gram Tomato, cut into 8 wedges

100 ml vegetable or pasta stock

1 tbsp Chopped parsley

Directions:

Heat the oven to 200C / gas mark 6.

Start using the hot celery. Heat a skillet over moderate-low heat, then add the olive oil, then the garlic, onion, ginger, celery, and peppermint. Fry lightly for two-three minutes until softened but not colored, you can add the curry powder and cook for a further minute.

Insert the berries afterward, your lentils and stock, and simmer for 10 seconds. You might choose to increase or reduce the cooking time according to how crunchy you'd like your own sausage.

Meanwhile, mix the garlic olive oil and lemon juice and then rub the salmon. # Set on the baking dish and cook 8--10 seconds.

In order to complete, stir the skillet throughout the celery and function with the salmon.

Nutrition:

Calories: 515 Cal

Fat: 28.51 g

Protein: 148.52 g

Sugar: 77.9 g

28coronation Steak Salad-Sirtfood Recipes

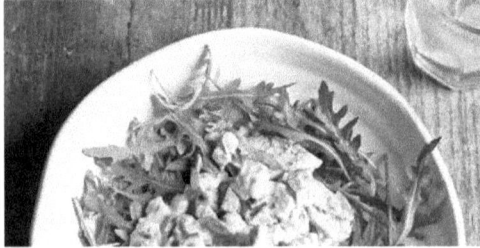

Preparation Time: 10 minutes

Cooking Time: 0 minutes

Servings: 3

Ingredients:

75 G Natural yogurts

Juice Of 1/4 of a lemon

1 Tsp Coriander, sliced

1 Tsp Ground turmeric

1/2 Tsp darkened curry powder

100 G Cooked chicken, cut to bite-sized pieces

6 Walnut halves, finely chopped

1 Medjool date, finely chopped

20 G Crimson pumpkin, diced

1 Bird's eye illuminates

40 Gram Rocket, to function

Directions:

Mix The lemon, carrot juice, spices, and coriander together in a bowl. Add all of the remaining ingredients and serve on a bed of this rocket.

Nutrition:

Calories: 528 Cal

Fat: 50.14 g

Protein: 23 8g

Sugar: 34.7 g

29sesame Chicken Salad

Preparation Time: 10 minutes

Cooking Time: 12 minutes

Servings: 2

Ingredients:

1 tbsp sesame seeds

One cucumber, peeled, half-long, desired with a teaspoon and 100 g sliced baby kale, roughly chopped

60 g pak choi, very finely shredded

1⁄2 red onion, very finely sliced

A big handful (20 g) of petroleum, chopped

150 g cooked chicken, shredded

For dressing:

1 tbsp of extra virgin olive oil

1 tsp of sesame oil

One lime juice

1 tsp of sugar

2 tsp of soy sauce

Directions:

In A hot frying pan, the sesame seeds toast for 2 minutes until lightly browned and fragrant. Move to a cold plate.

Combine the olive oil, sesame oil, lime juice, honey, and soy sauce in a small bowl to make a dressing.

In a large bowl, put the cucumber, the kale, the pak choi, the red onion, and the parsley and combine gently. Pour over the sauce, then again blend.

Divide the salad with the shredded chicken between two plates, and top. Just before eating, brush over the sesame seeds.

Nutrition:

Calories: 304 Cal

Fat: 95.86 g

Protein: 74.38 g

Sugar: 6.37 g

30sirt Food Miso-Marinated Cod With Stir-Fried Greens & Sesame-Sirtfoods Recipes

Preparation Time: 10 minutes

Cooking Time: 10 minutes

Servings: 2

Ingredients:

20g miso

1 tbsp mirin

1 tbsp of extra virgin olive oil

200 g of skinless cod fillet

20 g of red onion, sliced

40 g of celery, sliced

One garlic clove, finely chopped

One bird's eye chili, finely chopped

1 tsp of fresh ginger

60 g of green beans

50 g of kale, roughly chopped

1 tsp of sesame seeds

5 g of parsley, roughly chopped

1 tbsp of tamari

30 g of buckwheat

1 tsp of turmeric

Directions:

Mix the miso, mirin, and oil in a tablespoon. Rub the cod all over and leave for 30 minutes to marinate. Bake the cod for about 10 minutes.

Meanwhile, heat the remaining oil to a large frying pan or wok. Stir-fry the onion for a few minutes, then add the celery, garlic, chili, ginger, green beans, and kale. Toss and fry until the kale is cooked through and tender. To aid the cooking process, you might need to add a little water to the pan. Cook the buckwheat with the turmeric for 3 minutes according to the directions on the packet. To the stir-fry, add the sesame seeds, parsley, and tamari and serve with the greens and fish.

Nutrition:

Calories: 355 Cal

Fat: 10.87 g

Protein: 40.31 g

Sugar: 5.17 g

31Moong Dahl

Preparation Time: 10 minutes

Cooking Time: 15 minutes

Servings: 5

Ingredients:

300g/10 of split mung beans (Moong Dahl)–preferably soaked for a few hours

600ml/1pt water

Two tbsp/30 g olive oil, butter or ghee

One red onion, finely chopped

1-2 tsp of coriander seeds

1-2 tsp of cumin seeds

2-4 tsp of fresh ginger, chopped

1-2 tsp of turmeric

1/4 tsp of cayenne pepper–more if you want it spicy

Salt & black pepper to taste

Directions:

Drain and rinse split mung beans. Place in a casserole, and cover with water. Bring to the boil and skim off any moisture that comes up. Turn the heat down, cover and simmer.

In a heavy-bottomed pan, dry fry the coriander and cumin seeds until they begin to pop. Grind them in a mortar and pestle.

Attach the ground spices and the ginger, turmeric, and cayenne pepper to the onions. Cook in a couple of minutes.

Nutrition:

Calories: 430 Cal

Fat: 32.1 g

Protein: 12.37 g

Sugar: 17.3 g

Chapter 11: Fish Recipes

32baked Fish With Mushroom-Wine Sauce

Preparation Time: 10 minutes

Cooking Time: 10 minutes

Servings: 2

Ingredients:

Cod, haddock, or scrod work equally well in this dish.

2 teaspoons margarine

1 cup chopped mushrooms

2 tablespoons lemon juice

1 small garlic clove, minced Dash each salt and pepper

10 ounces fish fillets

1/4 cup each chopped scallions (green onions) and dry vermouth

1 tablespoon chopped fresh parsley(optional)

Directions:

Preheat oven to 400°F. In small skillet heat margarine until bubbly and hot; add mushrooms, lemon juice, garlic, and seasonings and sauté over high heat, occasionally stirring, until most of the liquid has evaporated.

Place fish in 1-quart casserole and top with mushroom mixture, scallions, and vermouth; bake until fish is opaque and flakes easily when tested with a fork, about 10 minutes. If desired, sprinkle with parsley just before serving.

Nutrition:

Calories: 197 Cal

Fat: 4 g

Protein: 26 g

Sugar: 2.73 g

33baked Cod Livornese

Preparation Time:

Cooking Time:

Servings: 2

Ingredients:

2 teaspoons olive oil

1/4 cup chopped onion

1 garlic clove, minced

1/2 cup chopped mushrooms

1/4 cup white wine

1/2 cup canned Italian tomatoes, chopped

1/4 teaspoon each basil leaves, oregano leaves, and salt Dash pepper

10 ounces cod fillets

2 teaspoons grated Parmesan cheese

1 tablespoon chopped fresh parsley

Directions:

Preheat oven to 400°F. In 10-inch skillet heat oil; add onion and garlic and sauté until onion is translucent about 1 minute.

Add mushrooms and cook until mushrooms are just tender about 2 minutes; add the wine and bring to a boil. Add tomatoes and seasonings and cook, occasionally stirring, until sauce thickens, about 2 minutes.

In shallow 1-quart flameproof casserole, arrange fillets and top with sauce; sprinkle with cheese and bake until fish flakes easily at the touch of a fork, 15 to 20 minutes.

Using slotted pancake turner, carefully remove fish from casserole to serving platter; keep fish warm. Place the casserole over medium heat and cook remaining pan juices until reduced and thickened, about 2 minutes; pour over fish and serve sprinkled with parsley.

Nutrition:

Calories: 213 Cal

Fat: 6 g

Protein: 27 g

Sugar: 5.96 g

34salmon With Asparagus Sauce

Preparation Time: 10 minutes

Cooking Time: 15 minutes

Servings: 2

Ingredients:

2 teaspoons olive oil

1 tablespoon minced shallots

1 garlic clove, minced

1/2 cup cooked chopped asparagus

1/2 teaspoon salt, divided

1/4 teaspoon white pepper, divided

2 teaspoons mayonnaise

1/4 teaspoon Dijon-style mustard

1 salmon fillet,10 ounces

1/4 cup dry white wine

2 teaspoons grated Parmesan cheese

Directions:

In 9-inch skillet heat oil, add shallots and garlic and sauté until shallots are translucent, being careful not to burn the garlic.

Transfer shallot mixture to blender container. Add asparagus, 1/4 teaspoon salt, and 1/2 teaspoon pepper and process until smooth; set aside.

Preheat oven to 400°F. in a small bowl combine mayonnaise and mustard; spread on fillet and sprinkle with remaining 1/4 teaspoon salt and 1/2 teaspoon pepper. Transfer salmon to 8 x 8 x 2-inch nonstick baking pan; add the wine and bake until fish flakes easily when tested with a fork, about 15 minutes (exact timing will depend upon the thickness of fillet).

Remove pan from oven and turn oven control to broil. Spread asparagus puree over fish and sprinkle with cheese. Broil just until heated through.

Nutrition:

Calories: 431 Cal

Fat: 28 g

Protein: 34 g

Sugar: 2.22 g

35Batter and Fish
Preparation Time: 10 minutes

Cooking Time: 10 minutes

Servings: 2

Ingredients:

3 tablespoons all-purpose flour

1/4 teaspoon double-acting baking powder

1/2s teaspoon salt

3 tablespoons water

10 ounces scrod fillets, cut into 1-inch pieces

1 tablespoon plus 1 teaspoon vegetable oil

Sweet 'n' Sour Medley

1/22 cup diagonally sliced carrot (thin slices)

1/4 cup water

1/2 cup canned pineapple chunks (no sugar added), drain and reserve juice

1/4 cup each diced red and green bell peppers

2 teaspoons each firmly packed

brown sugar and teriyaki sauce

1 teaspoon each cornstarch and rice wine vinegar

1/2 teaspoon salt

Directions:

To Prepare Sweet 'n' Sour Medley: In 1-quart saucepan combine carrot and water; bring to a boil. Reduce heat, cover, and let simmer until carrot slices are tender about 3 minutes; stir in pineapple chunks and red and green peppers and cook until mixture is heated. In measuring cup or small bowl combine reserved pineapple juice with remaining ingredients for sweet 'n' sour medley, stirring to dissolve cornstarch; pour over carrot mixture and cook, constantly stirring, until mixture thickens and is thoroughly heated. Set aside.

To Prepare Fish: In a small bowl, using a fork, combine dry ingredients, add water and stir until batter is smooth. Add fish pieces to the batter and turn until thoroughly coated.

In 10-inch nonstick skillet heat oil over medium-high heat; add fish and cook until golden brown on the bottom, 3 to 4 minutes. Carefully turn pieces over and cook until another side is browned; remove to a serving platter and top with warm sweet 'n' sour medley.

Nutrition:

Calories: 323 Cal

Fat: 11 g

Protein: 27 g

Sugar: 28.85 g

Chapter 12: Snacks

36the Sirtfood Juice

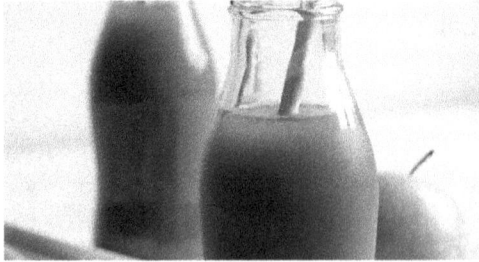

A good way to get started is with The Sirtfood Juice – so we've thrown this in the recipe to start you off as an extra bonus.

Preparation Time: 15 minutes

Cooking Time: 0 minutes

Servings: 1

Ingredients:

2 large handfuls (75 g) kale

a large handful (30 g) rocket

a very small handful (5 g) flat-leaf parsley

a very small handful (5 g) lovage leaves (optional)

2–3 large stalks (150 g) green celery, including its leaves

1⁄2 medium green beans.

Directions:

We notice juicers may really differ in their efficiency when juicing leafy vegetables, and before going on to the other ingredients, you will need to re-juice the remains. The target is to finish off the greens with about 50ml of water.

Now you can peel the lemon and even bring it through the juicer, but we find it much easier to squeeze the lemon in the juice by hand simply. You should have about 250ml of juice in total by this point, maybe a little bit more. It's only when the juice is made and ready to serve that you add the green tea matcha.

In a bowl, pour a small amount of water, then add the matcha, and stir vigorously with a fork or tablespoon. In the first two drinks of the day, we only use matcha, as it contains small levels of caffeine (the same content as a regular teacup). If drunk late. Once the matcha is dissolved, add the remainder of the drink, it can keep them awake for people not used to it.

Give it a swirl end; then, your juice is ready to drink. Free to top up with plain tea, as you want.

Nutrition:

Calories: 12 Cal

Fat: 0.56 g

Protein: 0.34 g

Sugar: 0.5 g

37Sirt Muesli

Simply mix the dry ingredients and place them in an airtight container if you want to make this in bulk or prepare it the night before. The following day all you need to do is add the strawberries and yogurt, and it's ready to go.

Preparation Time: 15 minutes

Cooking Time: 0 minutes

Servings: 2

Ingredients:

20 g buckwheat flakes

10 g buckwheat puffs

15 g coconut flakes or desiccated coconut

40 g Medjool dates, pitted and chopped

15 g walnuts, chopped

10 g cocoa nibs

100 g strawberries, hulled and chopped

100 g plain Greek yogurt (or vegan substitute, such as soya or coconut yogurt)

Directions:

Mix all the above-mentioned ingredients together (leave the strawberries and yogurt aside).

Nutrition:

Calories: 368 Cal

Fat: 11.05 g

Protein: 16.54 g

Sugar: 39.54 g

38aromatic Chicken Breast With Kale And Red Onions And A Tomato And Chili Salsa

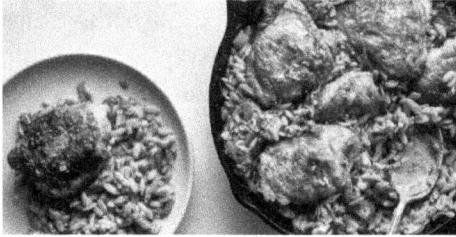

Preparation Time: 15 minutes

Cooking Time: 15 minutes

Servings: 3

Ingredients:

120 g skinless, boneless chicken breast

2 tsp ground turmeric

juice of 1⁄4 lemon

1 tbsp extra virgin olive oil

50 g kale, chopped

20 g red onion, sliced

1 tsp chopped fresh ginger

50 g buckwheat

For salsa

130 g tomato (about 1)

1 bird's eye chili, finely chopped

1 tbsp capers, finely chopped

5 g parsley, finely chopped

1⁄4 lemon juice

Directions:

Mix with the chili, capers, lemon juice, and parsley. You could put it all in a blender, but the end result is a bit different.

Oven heat to 220oC / gas 7. Marinate the chicken breast with the turmeric, lemon juice and a little oil in 1 tablespoon. Heat an ovenproof frying pan until hot, then add the marinated chicken and cook on each side for about a minute or so until pale golden, then transfer to the oven (place on a baking tray if your pan is not ovenproof) for 8-10 minutes or until cooked through. Remove from the oven, cover with foil, and allow to rest before serving for 5 minutes.

Meanwhile, boil the kale for 5 minutes in a steamer. In a little oil, fry the red onions and ginger until soft but not colored, then add the cooked kale and fry for another minute. Cook the buckwheat with the remaining turmeric teaspoon in accordance with the packet instructions. Serve with chicken, tomatoes, and salsa.

Nutrition:

Calories: 341 Cal

Fat: 10.74 g

Protein: 33.86 g

Sugar: 5.31 g

39sirtfood Bites

Preparation Time: 10 minutes

Cooking Time: 10 minutes

Servings: 12

Ingredients:

120 g walnuts

30 g dark chocolate (85% solid cocoa), broken into pieces; or cocoa nibs

250 g Medjool dates, pitted

1 tbsp cocoa powder

1 tbsp turmeric ground

1 tbsp extra virgin olive oil scraped seeds

1 vanilla pod or 1 tsp vanilla extract

2 tbsp water

Directions:

Put the walnuts and chocolate in a food processor and process until you have a food processor.

Add all the remaining ingredients except water and combine until the mixture forms a disc. Depending on the consistency of the mixture, you may or may not have to add the water; you don't want it to be too sticky.

Shape the mixture into bite-sized balls using your hands and refrigerate for at least 1 hour in an airtight container before eating them. In some more cocoa or desiccated coconut, you could roll some of the balls to achieve a different finish if you like. They can keep it in your fridge for up to 1 week.

Nutrition:

Calories: 698 Cal

Fat: 98.43 g

Protein: 27.08 g

Sugar: 177.43 g

Sugar: 100 g

40lemon Ricotta Cookies With Lemon Glaze

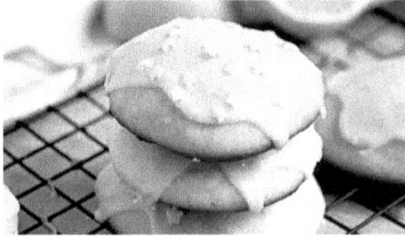

Preparation Time: 20 minutes

Cooking Time: 25 minutes

Servings: 12

Ingredients:

2 1/2 cups all-purpose flour

1 tsp baking powder

1 tsp salt

1 tbsp unsalted butter softened

2 cups of sugar

2 capsules

1 teaspoon (15-ounce) container whole-milk ricotta cheese

3 tbsp lemon juice

1 lemon, zested

Glaze:

11/2 cups powdered sugar

3 tbsp lemon juice

1 lemon, zested

Directions:

Pre heats the oven to 375 degrees F.

In a medium bowl, mix the flour, baking powder, and salt. Set aside.

From the big bowl, blend the butter and the sugar levels. With an electric mixer, beat the sugar and butter until light and fluffy, about three minutes. Add the eggs1 at a time, beating until incorporated.

Insert the ricotta cheese, lemon juice, and lemon zest. Beat to blend. Stir in the dry skin.

Line two baking sheets with parchment paper. Spoon the dough (approximately 2 tablespoons of each cookie) on the baking sheets. Bake for fifteen minutes, until slightly golden at the borders. Remove from the oven and let the biscuits remaining baking sheet for about 20 minutes.

Glaze:

Combine the powdered sugar lemon juice and lemon peel in a small bowl and then stir until smooth. Spoon approximately 1/2-tsp on each cookie and make use of the back of the spoon to disperse lightly. Allow glaze to harden for approximately two hours. Pack the biscuits to a decorative jar.

Nutrition:

Calories: 298 Cal

Fat: 11.9 g

Protein: 33.99 g

Sugar: 739 g

41home-Made Marshmallow Fluff

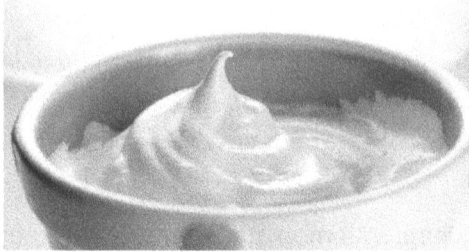

Preparation Time: 30 minutes

Cooking Time: 2 hours

Servings: 20

Ingredients:

3/4 cup sugar

1/2 cup light corn syrup

1/4 cup water

⅛ tsp salt

3 little egg whites egg whites

1/4 tsp cream of tartar

1 teaspoon 1/2 tsp vanilla infusion

Directions:

In a little pan, mix together sugar, corn syrup, salt, and water. Attach a candy thermometer into the side of this pan, which makes sure it will not touch the underside of the pan. Set aside.

From the bowl of a stand mixer, combine egg whites and cream of tartar. Begin to whip on medium speed with the whisk attachment.

Meanwhile, turn the burner on top and place the pan with the sugar mix onto heat. Allow mix into a boil and heat to 240 degrees, stirring periodically.

The aim is to find the egg whites whipped to soft peaks and also the sugar heated to 240 degrees at near the same moment. Simply stop stirring the egg whites once they hit soft peaks.

Once the sugar has already reached 240 amounts, turn noodle onto reducing. Insert a little quantity of the popular sugar mix and let it mix. Insert still another little sum of the sugar mix. Carry on adding mix slowly, and that means you never scramble the egg whites.

After all of the sugar was added into the egg whites, then turn the rate of this mixer and also keep overcoming concoction for around 79 minutes until the fluff remains glossy and stiff. In roughly the 5-minute mark, then add vanilla extract.

Use fluff immediately or store in an airtight container in the fridge for around two weeks

Nutrition:

Calories: 211 Cal

Fat: 29.51 g

Protein: 26.94 g

Sugar: 206 g

42guilt Totally Free Banana Ice Cream

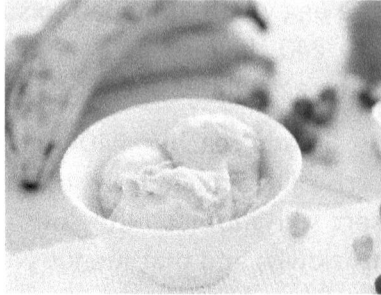

Preparation Time: 15 minutes

Cooking Time: 0 minutes

Servings: 3

Ingredients:

3 quite ripe banana - peeled and rooted

a couple of chocolate chips

two Tbsp skim milk

Directions:

Throw all ingredients into a food processor and blend until creamy.

Eat freeze and appreciate afterward.

Nutrition:

Calories: 706 Cal

Fat: 26.18 g

Protein: 12.6 g

Sugar: 78.75 g

43perfect Little Pb Snack Balls

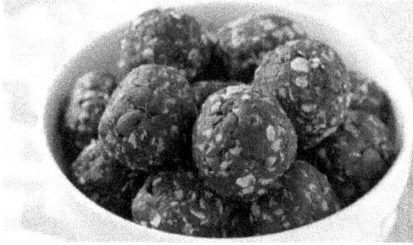

Preparation Time: 10 minutes

Cooking Time: 0 minutes

Servings: 15

Ingredients:

1/2 cup chunky peanut butter

3 Tbsp flax seeds

3 Tbsp wheat germ

1 Tbsp honey or agave

1/4 cup powder

Directions:

Blend dry ingredients and adding from the honey and peanut butter.

Mix well and roll into chunks and then conclude by rolling into wheatgerm.

Nutrition:

Calories: 117 Cal

Fat: 1.58 g

Protein: 4.15 g

Sugar: 2.68 g

44dark Chocolate Pretzel Cookies

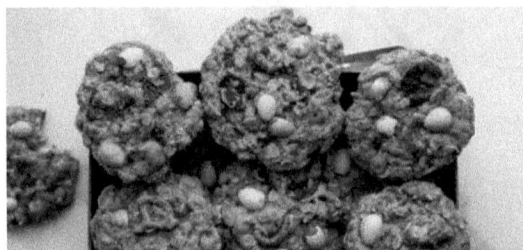

Preparation Time: 15 minutes

Cooking Time: 20 minutes

Servings: 20

Ingredients:

1 cup yogurt

1/2 tsp baking soda

1/4 teaspoon salt

1/4 tsp cinnamon

4 Tbsp butter softened

1/3 cup brown sugar

1 egg

1/2 tsp vanilla

1/2 cup dark chocolate chips

1/2 cup pretzels chopped

Directions:

Pre Heat oven to 350 degrees.

At a medium bowl, whisk together the sugar, butter, vanilla, and egg.

In another bowl, stir together the flour, baking soda, and salt.

Stir the bread mixture in using all the moist components, along with the chocolate chips and pretzels until just blended.

Drop large spoonful of dough on an unlined baking sheet.

Bake for 15-17 minutes, or until the bottoms are somewhat all crispy.

Allow cooling on a wire rack.

Nutrition:

Calories: 1017 Cal

Fat: 65.46 g

Protein: 22.74 g

Sugar: 44.8 g

45thai Nut Mix

Preparation Time: 30 minutes

Cooking Time: 20 minutes

Servings: 4

Ingredients:

½ cup walnuts

½ cup coconut flakes

½ tsp soy sauce

1 tsp honey

1 pinch of cayenne pepper

1 dash of lime juice

Directions:

Add the above ingredients to a bowl, toss the nuts to coat, and place on a baking sheet, lined with parchment paper. Cook at 250 F for 15-20 minutes, checking as not to burn, but lightly toasted.

Remove from oven. Cool first before eating.

Nutrition:

Calories: 496 Cal

Fat: 38.49 g

Protein: 7.82 g

Sugar: 23.75 g

Chapter 13: Dinner

46bang-Bang Chicken Noodle Stir-Fry Recipe

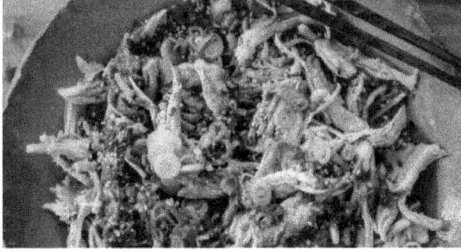

Preparation Time: 15 minutes

Cooking Time: 25 minutes

Servings: 10

Ingredients:

1 tablespoon sunflower oil

750g package chicken thighs, boned, any surplus skin trimmed

250g frozen chopped mixed peppers

Inch courgetti, peeled into ribbons, seeded center chopped

1 chicken stock cube

250g pack moderate egg yolks

4 garlic cloves, finely chopped

1/2 tsp crushed chilies, and additional to serve (optional)

4 tablespoons reduced-salt soy sauce

2 tsp caster sugar

1 lime, zested, 1/2 juiced, 1/2 slice into wedges to function

Directions:

Heat the oil in a skillet on a medium-low warmth. Fry the chicken skin-side down to 10 mins or until your skin is emptied. Flip and simmer for 10 mins, or until cooked. Transfer to a plate cover loosely with foil.

Reheat the wok over a high temperature, add the peppers and sliced courgette; simmer for 5 mins. Meanwhile, bring a bowl of water to the boil, then crumble in the stock block, adding the noodles. Simmer for 45 mins until cooked, then drain well.

Insert the garlic and crushed chilies into the wok; simmer for two mins. In a bowl, mix the soy sugar and the lime juice and zest. Enhance the wok, bubble 2 mins; you can add the courgette noodles and ribbons. Toss with tongs to coat in the sauce.

Cut the chicken into pieces. Divide the noodles between 4 bowls and top with the chicken. Serve with the lime wedges along with extra crushed chilies, in case you prefer.

Nutrition:

Calories: 367 Cal

Fat: 236.38 g

Protein: 318.56 g

Sugar: 31.55 g

47pesto Salmon Pasta Noodles Recipe

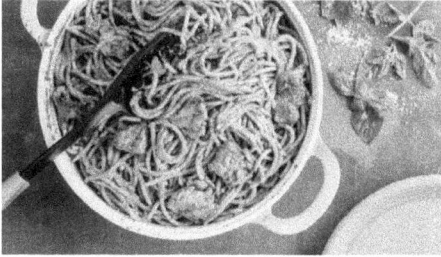

Preparation Time: 15 minutes

Cooking Time: 25 minutes

Servings: 3

Ingredients:

350g penne

2 x 212g tins cherry salmon, drained

1 lemon, zested and juiced

190g jar green pesto

250g package cherry tomatoes halved

100g bunch spring onions, finely chopped

125g package reduced-fat mozzarella

Directions:

Pre heats the oven to Windows 7, 220°C, buff 200°C. Boil the pasta for 5 mins. Drain, reserving 100ml drinking water.

Meanwhile, at a 2ltr ovenproof dish, then mix the salmon, lemon zest, and juice, then pesto (booking 2 tablespoons) berries and half of the spring onions; season.

105

Mix the pasta and reserved cooking water to the dish. Mix the allowed pesto using 1 tablespoon water and then drizzle on the pasta. Gently within the mozzarella, top with the rest of the spring onions and bake for 25 mins until golden.

Nutrition:

Calories: 669 Cal

Fat: 58.18 g

Protein: 59.11 g

Sugar: 56.1 g

48sri Lankan-Style Sweet Potato Curry Recipe

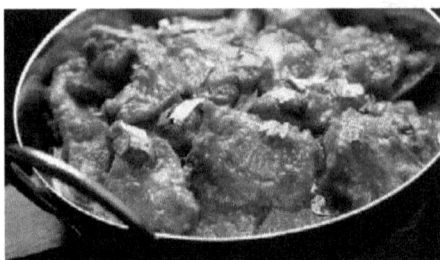

Preparation Time: 20 minutes

Cooking Time: 40 minutes

Servings: 6

Ingredients:

1/2 onion, roughly sliced

3 garlic cloves, roughly sliced

25g sliced ginger, chopped and peeled

15g fresh coriander stalks and leaves split leaves sliced

two 1/2 tablespoon moderate tikka curry powder

60g package cashew nuts

1 tablespoon olive oil

500g Redmere Farms sweet potatoes, peeled and cut into 3cm balls

400ml tin Isle Sun Coconut-milk

1/2 vegetable stock block, created as much as 300ml

200g Grower's Harvest long-grain rice

300g frozen green beans

150g Redmere Farms lettuce

1 Suntrail Farms lemon, 1/2 juiced, 1/2 cut into wedges to function

Directions:

Set the onion, ginger, garlic, coriander stalks, tikka powder along with half of the cashew nuts in a food processor. Insert 2 tablespoons water and blitz to a chunky paste.

At a large skillet, warm the oil over moderate heat. Insert the paste and cook, stirring for 5 mins. Bring the sweet potatoes, stir, then pour into the coconut milk and stock. Bring to the simmer and boil for 25-35 mins before the sweet potatoes are tender.

Meanwhile, cook the rice pack directions. Toast the rest of the cashews at a dry skillet.

Sti-R the beans into the curry and then simmer for two mins. Insert the lettuce in handfuls, allowing each to simmer before adding the following; simmer for 1 minute. Bring the lemon juice, to taste, & the majority of the coriander leaves. Scatter on the remaining coriander and cashews, then use the rice and lemon wedges.

Nutrition:

Calories: 544 Cal

Fat: 20 g

Protein: 36 g

Sugar: 14 g

49chicken Liver Along With Tomato Ragu Recipe

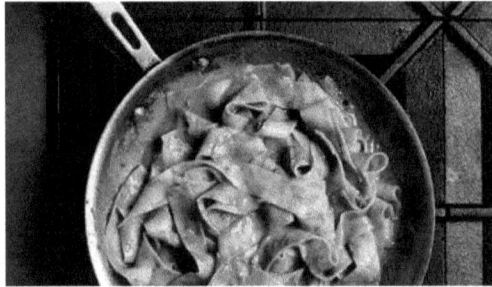

Preparation Time: 30 minutes

Cooking Time: 35 minutes

Servings: 3

Ingredients:

2 tablespoon olive oil

1 onion, finely chopped

2 carrots, scrubbed and simmer

4 garlic cloves, finely chopped

1/4 x 30g pack fresh ginger, stalks finely chopped, leaves ripped

380g package poultry livers, finely chopped, and almost any sinew removed and lost

400g tin Grower's Harvest chopped berries

1 chicken stock cube, created around 300ml

1/2 tsp caster sugar

300g penne

1/4 Suntrail Farms lemon, juiced

Directions:

Heat 1 tablespoon oil in a large skillet, over a low-medium heating system. Fry the onion and carrots to 10 mins, stirring periodically. Stir in the ginger and garlic pops and cook 2 mins more. Transfer into a bowl set aside.

Twist the pan into high heat and then add the oil. Bring the chicken livers and simmer for 5 mins until browned. Pour the onion mix to the pan and then stir in the tomatoes, sugar, and stock. Season bring to the boil, and then simmer for 20 mins until reduced and thickened, and also the liver is cooked through. Meanwhile, cook pasta to package Direction. Taste the ragu and put in a second pinch of sugar more seasoning, if needed. Put in a squeeze of lemon juice to taste and stir in two of the ripped basil leaves. Divide the pasta between four bowls, then spoon across the ragu and top with the rest of the basil.

Nutrition:

Calories: 3211 Cal

Fat: 114.52 g

Protein: 92.77 g

Sugar: 12 g

50minted Lamb With A Couscous Salad Recipe

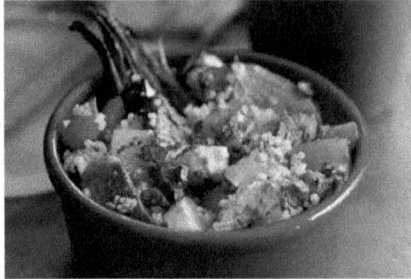

Preparation Time:

Cooking Time:

Servings: 5

Ingredients:

1/2 chicken stock block, composed to 125ml

30g pack refreshing flat-leaf parsley, sliced

3 mint sprigs, leaves picked and sliced

1 tablespoon olive oil

200g pack suspended BBQ minted lamb leg beans, De-frosted

200g lettuce berries, sliced

1/4 tsp, sliced

1 spring onion, sliced

pinch of ground cumin

1/2 lemon, zested and juiced

50g reduced-fat salad cheese

75g Cous-cous

Directions:

Place the couscous into a heatproof bowl and then pour on the inventory. Cover and set aside for 10 mins, then fluff with a fork and stir in the herbs.

Meanwhile, rub a little oil within the lamb steaks and season. Cook to package Direction, then slit.

Mix the tomatoes, cucumber and spring onion into the couscous with the oil, the cumin, and lemon juice and zest. Crumble on the salad and serve with the bunny.

Nutrition:

Calories: 463 Cal

Fat: 19 g

Protein: 33.8 g

Sugar: 11 g

51super-Speedy Prawn Risotto

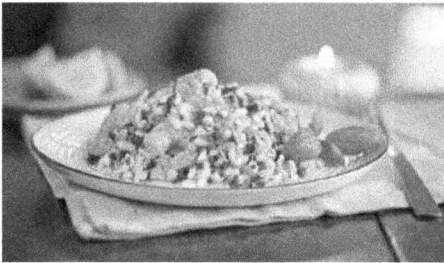

Preparation Time:

Cooking Time:

Servings: 4

Ingredients:

100g Diced Onion

Two X 250g packs whole-grain Rice & Quinoa

200g Frozen Garden Peas

Two x 150g packs Cooked and Peeled King Prawns

1/285g Tote watercress

Directions:

Heating 1 tablespoon coconut oil in a skillet on medium-high heat and then put in 100g Diced Onion; cook 5 mins. Insert 2 x 250g packs whole-grain Rice & Quinoa along with 175ml hot vegetable stock (or plain water), together side 200g suspended Garden Peas. Gently split using rice using a wooden spoon. Cover and cook 3 mins, stirring occasionally, you can add two x 150g packs Cooked and Peeled King Prawns. Cook for 12 mins before prawns, peas, and rice have been piping hot, and the majority of the liquid was consumed. Remove from heat. Chop 1/2 x 85g tote watercress and stir throughout; up to taste. Top with watercress leaves and pepper to function.

Nutrition:

Calories: 1077 Cal

Fat: 7.08 g

Protein: 40.1 g

Sugar: 34.01 g

Chapter 14: Desserts

52dark Chocolate Mousse [Vegan]

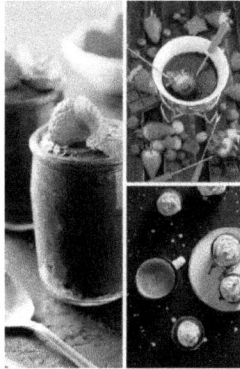

Delectable, smooth, sweet, calming. Those are just some of the adjectives that describe the enjoyment chocolate can bring to your life, which is why many of the dessert recipes to follow incorporate the high-quality Sirtfood ingredient. This particular recipe might be one of the most decadent indulgences you'll ever eat that you don't have to feel guilty about.

Preparation Time: 10 minutes

Cooking Time: 2 hours plus cooling time

Servings: 4

Ingredients:

1 (16 ounce) package silken tofu, drained

½ cup pure maple syrup

1 teaspoon pure vanilla extract

¼ cup soymilk

½ cup unsweetened cocoa powder

Mint leaves (optional and highly encouraged)

Directions:

Place tofu, maple syrup and vanilla in a food processor or blender. Process until well blended.

Add remaining ingredients and process until mixture is fully blended.

Pour into small dessert cups or espresso cups. Chill for at least 2 hours.

Nutrition:

Calories: 544 Cal

Fat: 6.95 g

Protein: 8.82 g

Sugar: 99.75 g

53loaded Chocolate Fudge

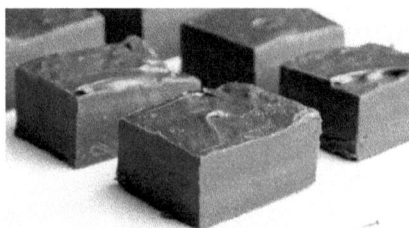

Many fudge recipes use sugar-loaded dairy products, which may taste good, but they're doing nothing for your health.

This loaded chocolate fudge still has sugar, but it's all natural and full of vitamins and antioxidants as well. Moderate the size of your bites but enjoy this fudge with the knowledge that you're still eating healthy ingredients.

Preparation Time: 10 minutes

Cooking Time: 1 hour plus cooling time

Servings: 16

Ingredients:

1 cup Medjool dates, chopped

2 tablespoons coconut oil, melted

1/2 cup peanut butter

¼ cup of unsweetened cocoa powder

½ cup walnuts

1 teaspoon vanilla

Directions:

Soak the dates in warm water for 20 – 30 minutes

Lightly grease an 8" square baking pan with coconut oil.

Add dates, peanut butter, cocoa powder and vanilla to a food processer and blend until smooth.

Fold in walnuts.

Pack into the greased baking pan and put in your freezer for 1 hour or until fudge is solid and firm.

Cut into 16 or more bite-sized squares and store in semi-airtight container in refrigerator.

Nutrition:

Calories: 992 Cal

Fat: 79.21 g

Protein: 19.51 g

Sugar: 42.49 g

54chocolate Maple Walnuts

This is a super simple recipe that makes a great dinner party dessert that everyone can indulge in as much or as little as they personally choose. The maple syrup plays off the bitterness of the dark chocolate perfectly, and the walnuts provide just the right texture for your guests or family to sink their teeth into.

Preparation Time: 15 minutes

Cooking Time: 30 minutes cooling time

Servings: 2 cups od candied walnuts

Ingredients:

½ cup pure maple syrup, divided

2 cups raw, whole walnuts

5 squares of dark chocolate, at least 85%

1 ½ tablespoons coconut oil, melted

1 tablespoonful of water

Sifted icing sugar

1 teaspoonful of vanilla extract

Directions:

Line a large baking sheet with parchment paper.

In a medium to large skillet, combine the walnuts and ¼ cup of maple syrup and cook over medium heat, stirring continuously, until walnuts are completely covered with syrup and golden in color, about 3 – 5 minutes.

Pour the walnuts onto the parchment paper and separate into individual pieces with a fork. Allow to cool completely, at least 15 minutes.

In the meantime, melt the chocolate in a double boiler with the coconut oil. Add the remaining maple syrup and stir until thoroughly combined.

When walnuts are cooled, transfer them to a glass bowl and pour the melted chocolate syrup over top. Use a silicone spatula to mix until walnuts are completely covered gently.

Transfer back to the parchment paper lined baking sheet and, once again, separate each of the nuts with a fork.

Place the nuts in the fridge for 10 minutes or the freezer for 3 – 5 minutes, until chocolate has completely set.

Store in an airtight bag in your fridge.

Nutrition:

Calories: 2033 Cal

Fat: 124.83 g

Protein: 24.43 g

Sugar: 197.74 g

55matcha And Chocolate Dipped Strawberries

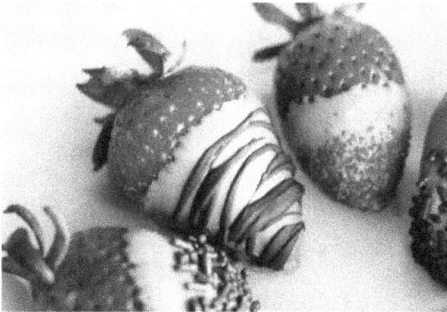

Chocolate dipped strawberries are possibly one of the most romantic desserts of all time. They're also great for warm summer evenings when you're craving something sweet but don't want a heavy cake or pudding. Eating them any other evening of the year is also just right. You can't go wrong.

Preparation Time: 25 minutes

Cooking Time: 25 minutes

Servings: 4 - 6

Ingredients:

4 tablespoons cocoa butter

4 squares of dark chocolate, at least 85%

¼ cup coconut oil

1 teaspoon Matcha green tea powder

20 – 25 large whole strawberries, stems on

Directions:

Melt cocoa butter, dark chocolate, coconut oil, and Matcha in a double boiler until nearly smooth.

Remove from heat and continue stirring until chocolate is completely melted.

Pour into a large glass bowl and stir constantly until the chocolate thickens and starts to lose its sheen, about 2 - 5 minutes.

Working one at a time, hold the strawberries by stems and dip into chocolate matcha mixture to coat. Let excess drip back into bowl.

Place on a parchment-lined baking sheet and chill dipped berries in the fridge until shell is set, 20–25 minutes.

You may need to reheat matcha mixture if it starts to set before you have dipped all the berries.

Nutrition:

Calories: 992 Cal

Fat: 101.65 g

Protein: 2.9 g

Sugar: 17.64 g

Chapter 15: Solid Food Recipes

56chicken With Red Onion And Black Cabbage

Preparation Time: 10 minutes

Cooking Time: 20 minutes

Servings: 6

Ingredients:

120g of chicken breast

130g of tomatoes

1 chili pepper

1 tablespoon of capers

5g of parsley

lemon juice

2 tbsp. Extra virgin olive oil

2 teaspoons of turmeric

50g of cabbage

20g of red onion

1 teaspoon fresh ginger

50g of buckwheat

Directions:

Marinate the chicken breast for 10 minutes with 1/4 of lemon juice, 1 tablespoon of extra virgin olive oil and 1 teaspoon of turmeric powder.

Cut 130g of chopped tomatoes, remove the inside, season with Bird's Eye pepper, 1 tablespoon of capers, 1 teaspoon of turmeric and one of extra virgin olive oil, 1/4 of lemon juice and 5g of parsley chopped.

Fry the chicken breast, dripped from the marinade, on a high flame for one minute on each side, then put it in the oven for about 10 minutes at 220 ° C.

Let it rest covered with aluminum foil.

Steam the chopped kale for 5 minutes.

Sauté a red onion, a teaspoon of grated fresh ginger and a teaspoon of extra virgin olive oil; add the cooked cabbage and cook for a minute on the fire.

Boil the buckwheat with a teaspoon of turmeric, drain and serve with chicken, tomatoes and chopped cabbage.

Nutrition:

Calories: 456 Cal

Fat: 24.28 g

Protein: 31.24 g

Sugar: 7.18 g

57buckwheat Salad

Buckwheat salad is a tasty first course, also excellent cold and gluten-free. It can be customized with the ingredients you prefer and never disappoints. Here is the recipe.

Preparation Time: 15 minutes

Cooking Time: 25 minutes

Servings: 4

Ingredients:

150g of buckwheat

150g of frozen beans (or fresh if in season)

1 courgette

1 carrot

1 clove of garlic

20g of salted capers

1 handful of sesame seeds (or sunflower)

Some basil leaves

1 teaspoon hot pepper

1 teaspoon balsamic vinegar to taste

Extra virgin olive oil to taste

Salt to taste.

Directions:

You cook!

First, blanch the beans in abundant salted water until they are cooked but al dente. Peel and cut the carrot into cubes half a centimeter thick. Do the same with courgette.

Cook the vegetables.

In a non-stick pan, heat a drizzle of extra virgin olive oil with the garlic clove. As soon as it has taken a little color and flavored the oil, remove it and add the chopped carrots. Cook for about 5 minutes, then add the courgettes and cook on a high flame for another 10 minutes, being careful not to burn the vegetables. A few minutes after the end of cooking, add the broad beans and season with the chili pepper, capers, sesame seeds and coarsely chopped basil by hand. Stir to mix all the ingredients well and season with salt.

Cook the wheat.

Boil the buckwheat in abundant salted water, then drain it al dente and season it with the vegetables. Add the balsamic vinegar and mix before serving.

Buckwheat salad can be kept in an airtight container and in the refrigerator for a couple of days.

Nutrition:

Calories: 243 Cal

Fat: 3.47 g

Protein: 10.05 g

Sugar: 7.76 g

Chapter 16: Special Sirtfood Recipes

58mocha Chocolate Mousse

Everybody appreciates chocolate mousse and this one has a brilliant light and breezy surface.

Preparation Time: 35 minutes

Cooking Time: 2 hours

Servings: 4-6

Ingredients:

250g dim chocolate (85% cocoa solids)

6 medium unfenced eggs, isolated

4 tbsp solid dark espresso

4 tbsp almond milk

Chocolate espresso beans, to enrich

Directions:

Soften the chocolate in a huge bowl set over a skillet of delicately stewing water, ensuring the base of the bowl doesn't contact the water. Expel the bowl from the heat and leave the dissolved chocolate to cool to room temperature.

When the softened chocolate is at room temperature, race in the egg yolks each in turn and afterward tenderly overlap in the espresso and almond milk.

Utilizing a hand-held electric blender, whisk the egg whites until firm pinnacles structure, at that point blend several tablespoons into the chocolate blend to release it. Delicately overlap in the rest of, an enormous metal spoon.

Move the mousse to singular glasses and smooth the surface. Spread with stick film and chill for in any event 2 hours, preferably medium-term. Enliven with chocolate espresso beans before serving.

Nutrition:

Calories: 112 Cal

Fat: 29.89 g

Protein: 40.3 g

Sugar: 128.13 g

59buckwheat Superfood Muesli

Preparation Time: 10 minutes

Cooking Time: 0 minutes

Servings: 2

Ingredients:

20g buckwheat pieces

10g buckwheat puffs

15g coconut pieces or parched coconut

40g Medjool dates, hollowed and cleaved

15g walnuts, cleaved

10g cocoa nibs

100g strawberries, hulled and cleaved

100g plain Greek yogurt (or veggie lover elective, for example, soy or coconut yogurt)

Directions:

Blend the entirety of the above Ingredients: together (forget about the strawberries and yogurt if not serving straight away).

NOTES

In the event that you need to make this in mass or set it up the prior night, just join the dry Ingredients: and store it in an impermeable holder. All you have to do the following day is include the strawberries and yogurt and it is all set.

Nutrition:

Calories: 486 Cal

Fat: 16.96 g

Protein: 22.05 g

Sugar: 37.37 g

60buckwheat Pancakes With Strawberries, Dark Chocolate Sauce And Crushed Walnuts-

Preparation Time: 5 minutes

Cooking Time: 15 minutes

Servings: 6 to 8 flapjacks, contingent upon the size.

Ingredients:

or the flapjacks you will require:

350ml milk

150g buckwheat flour

1 huge egg

1 tbsp additional virgin olive oil, for cooking

For the chocolate sauce

100g dull chocolate (85 percent cocoa solids)

85ml milk

1 tbsp twofold cream

1 tbsp additional virgin olive oil

To serve

400g strawberries, hulled and cleaved

100g walnuts, cleaved

Directions:

To make the hotcake player, place the entirety of the Ingredients: separated from the olive oil in a blender and mix until you have a smooth hitter. It ought not to be excessively thick or excessively runny. (You can store any abundance hitter in a water/air proof holder for as long as 5 days in your cooler. Make certain to blend a long time before utilizing once more.)

To make the chocolate sauce, soften the chocolate in a heatproof bowl over a container of stewing water. When dissolved, blend in the milk, whisking completely and afterward include the twofold cream and olive oil. You can keep the sauce warm by leaving the water in the dish stewing on an exceptionally low heat until your flapjacks are prepared.

To make the flapjacks heat a substantial bottomed griddle until it begins to smoke, at that point include the olive oil.

Empty a portion of the player into the focal point of the container, at that point tip the overabundance hitter around it until you have secured the entire surface, you may need to add somewhat more player to accomplish this. You will just need to cook the hotcake for 1 moment or so on each side if your dish is sufficiently hot.

When you can see it going dark colored around the edges utilize a spatula to release the flapjack around its edge, at that point flip it over. Attempt to flip in one activity to abstain from breaking it.

Cook for a further moment or so on the opposite side and move to a plate.

Spot a few strawberries in the middle and move up the flapjack. Proceed until you have made the same number of flapjacks as required.

Spoon over a liberal measure of sauce and sprinkle over some slashed walnuts.

You may find that your first endeavors are excessively fat or self-destruct however once you discover the consistency of your player that works best for you and you get your method culminated you'll be making them like an expert. Careful discipline brings about promising results right now.

Nutrition:

Calories: 189 Cal

Fat: 104.23 g

Protein: 48.37 g

Sugar: 76.92 g

61blueberry Smoothie

This yogurt smoothie has a rich, velvety taste.

Preparation Time: 10 minutes

Cooking Time: 0 minutes

Servings: 2

Ingredients:

1 ready banana

100g blueberries

100g blackberries

2 tbsp regular yogurt

200ml milk

Directions:

Mix all the Ingredients: together until smooth.

Nutrition:

Calories: 199 Cal

Fat: 1.46 g

Protein: 3.02 g

Sugar: 41.59 g

Conclusion

Sirtfood diet program is an idea it is possible to embark on, but perhaps not merely for weight loss but also for several due procedures indoors and out human body posture.

The plan asserts that eating particular foods can trigger your "lean receptor" pathway and possess you losing seven pounds in 7 days. Foods such as ginseng, dark chocolate, and milk contain a natural compound called polyphenols which mimic the results of fasting and exercise. Strawberries, red onions, cinnamon, and garlic will also be powerful Sirtfoods. These foods can activate the sirtuin pathway to help activate weight reduction. The science seems appealing; however, the truth is there is very little research to backup these claims. Plus, the guaranteed speed of weight reduction from the very first week is quite quick and perhaps not in accord with the national institute of health safe fat loss recommendations of a couple of pounds each week.

The diet contains two stages:

Phase inch last for 7 days. For the initial 3 days, you only drink three Sirtfood green juices along with something meal full of Sirtfoods for an overall total of 1000 calories. On days four through seven you drink 2 green juices along with 2 meals for a total of 1,500 calories.

Phase two is really a 14day maintenance program, though it's created to your shed weight steadily (perhaps not sustain your present weight). Daily is composed of three balanced Sirtfood meals plus also one green juice.

Those 3 weeks, you are invited to keep on eating a diet full of Sirtfoods and drinking a green juice each day. You can discover several Sirtfood collection recipes and online on the Sirtfood site. 1 green juice recipe entirely on the Sirtfood internet site is made up of combination of spinach and other leafy vegetables greens, celery, carrot, green apple, ginger, lemon juice and

Matcha. Buckwheat and Lovage may also be things which can be advocated for used on your green juice. They diet urges that apples should be made in a juicer, not just a blender, therefore it tastes better.

Knowledge Is Power- The diet is still very recent, but useful information is still available, and much remains to be done as this diet is rapidly gaining popularity. You can also search the Internet for recipes, food options, nutrients, etc.

Follow The Rules - Sirtfood is guaranteed to get results if you follow the recommended diet and meals closely.

Put In Place The First "Restrictions" - If you want to get different results, you obviously have to "sacrifice" a little to get the full result of the Sirtfood diet. Do not worry; the first three days are the most difficult for this diet because there are calorie restrictions. However, rest assured that every day is easier. Although the restrictions imposed were not so strict for some who followed the diet, the reason was good meal planning. You will not be hungry with the Sirtfood diet if you choose carefully.

Always consult your health care professional before starting a diet or diet, especially if you have a current medical condition. This ensures that the diet does not counteract any medication that you have taken or that has affected your health. Don't worry; the Sirtfood diet is pretty safe.

Part 2

Chapter 1: What Is Sirtfood Diet?

The sirtfood diet depends on the possibility that specific nourishments actuate sirtuins in your body, which are particular proteins guessed to receive different rewards, from shielding cells in your body from aggravation to switching maturing. Nourishments permitted on the eating regimen incorporate green tea, dim chocolate, apples, organic citrus products, parsley, turmeric, kale, blueberries, tricks and red wine.

On the authority Sirt food diet site, defenders clarify that the eating regimen has two "simple" stages. Stage one is seven days with every day comprising of three sort food green juices and one dinner loaded up with sirtfoods — a sum of 1,000 calories. You may be somewhat less starving on days four through seven when you're permitted to expand your admission to 1,500 calories with two green juices and two dinners.

Stage two isn't significantly more encouraging. This stage goes on for about fourteen days, in which you are allowed to have three "adjusted" sirtfood-rich suppers every day notwithstanding your one extraordinary green juice. The objective during this time is to advance further weight reduction. While the advantages of sirtuins appear to be encouraging, the sirtfood diet is promoted up 'til now another approach to "shed seven pounds in seven days!" And you know at this point outrageous weight control plans simply don't work that way.

What seems like a tidbit lifted directly from a science fiction motion picture, a 'sirtfood' is nourishment high in sirtuin activators. Sirtuins are a sort of protein which shield the cells in our bodies from biting the dust or getting aggravated through sickness, however, investigate has likewise demonstrated they can help manage your digestion, increment muscle and consume fat.

Two big-name nutritionists working for a private exercise centre in the UK built up the Sirtfood Diet. They promote the eating routine as a regular new eating routine and wellbeing plan that works by turning on your "thin quality." This eating regimen depends on to inquire about on sirtuins (SIRTs), a gathering of seven proteins found in the body that has been appeared to control an assortment of capacities, including digestion, irritation and life expectancy. Specific individual plant mixes might have the option to expand the degree of these proteins in the body, and nourishments containing them have been named "sirtfoods."

Introduction:

The Sirtfood Diet book was first distributed in the U.K. in 2016. Be that as it may, the U.S. arrival of the book, coming this March, has started the greater interest in the arrangement. The eating routine started getting publicity when Adele debuted her slimmer figure at the Billboard Music Awards last May. Her coach, Pete Geracimo, is a huge aficionado of the eating routine and says the vocalist shed 30 pounds from following a Sirt food diet.

Sirtfoods are wealthy in supplements that actuate a supposed "thin quality" called sirtuin. As indicated by Goggins and Matten, the "thin quality" is initiated when a lack of vitality is made after you confine calories. Sirtuins got fascinating to the nourishment world in 2003 when specialists found that resveratrol, a compound found in red wine, had a similar impact on life range as calorie limitation however it was accomplished without diminishing admission.

In the 2015 pilot study (led by Goggins and Matten) testing the viability of sirtuins, the 39 members lost a normal of seven pounds in seven days. Those outcomes sound noteworthy, yet it's critical to understand this is a small example size concentrated over a brief timeframe. Weight reduction specialists additionally have their questions about the elevated guarantees. "The cases made are extremely theoretical and extrapolate from examines which were generally centred around basic life forms (like yeast) at the cell level. What occurs at the cell level doesn't mean what occurs in the human body at the large scale level," says Adrienne Youdim, M.D., the executive of the Center for Weight Loss and Nutrition in Beverly Hills, CA.

What nourishments are high in sirtuins?

The book contains a rundown of the leading 20 nourishments that are high in sirtuins, which sounds more like a drifting nourishment list than another, advanced eating routine. Models include arugula, chillies, espresso, green tea, Medjool dates, red wine, turmeric, pecans, and the wellbeing cognizant top pick kale. Dr Youdim takes note of that while the nourishments being advanced are stable, they won't advance weight reduction all alone.

The fundamental reason of the Sirtfood Diet is that sure nourishments, named "sirtfoods," can emulate the demonstrated advantages of caloric limitation and fasting by method for actuating sirtuins—proteins in the body (going from SIRT1 to SIRT7) that manage natural pathways, turn certain qualities on and off, and help shield cells from age-related decay. Enactment of SIRT1, for instance, has been appeared in some lab and creature concentrates on initiating the development of new mitochondria, expanding life length, and improve oxidative digestion, which may bolster weight reduction and support.

Since fasting and extreme caloric limitation is extremely hard (and frequently, not fitting), Goggins and Matten built up their dietary arrangement—concentrated on eating heaps of "sirtfoods"— as a more straightforward method to invigorate the body's sirtuin qualities (in some cases alluded to as "thin qualities") and in this way increase weight reduction and advance by and broad wellbeing.

What makes something a "sirtfood"?

Some "sirtfoods" that Goggins and Matten notice in their book incorporates green tea, berries, cocoa powder, turmeric, kale, onions, parsley, arugula, chillies, espresso, red wine, pecans, escapades, buckwheat, and olive oil. These nourishments contain explicit polyphenol mixes (quercetin, resveratrol, kaempferol, and so on.) that have, truth be told, been found in logical investigations to increment sirtuin action. Along these lines, right now, diet is at any rate to some degree dependent on science.

The issue, notwithstanding, is that these nourishments may not contain adequate degrees of these polyphenols to enact sirtuins in any meaningful manner. A large number of the examinations connecting polyphenol mixes to expanded sirtuin action have just been done on exceptionally focused types of these mixes.

How is the Sirtfood Diet organized?

The Sirtfood Diet is separated into two fundamental stages: Stage One goes on for seven days. For the initial three days, the eating regimen calls for devouring three sirtfood green juices and one dinner rich in sirtfoods—for an aggregate of 1,000 calories for each day. Days four through seven, each comprise of two green juices and two dinners—for a sum of 1,500 calories for every day. This is the piece of the arrangement wherein Goggins and Matten guarantee you can "shed seven pounds in seven days."

Stage Two is a 14-day upkeep stage intended to "assist you with getting more fit relentlessly." You can have three sirtfood-rich dinners in addition to one green juice for every day.

As indicated by Goggins and Matten, these two stages can be rehashed as frequently as you'd like for a weight reduction support. Following these underlying three weeks, you're urged to keep "sirtifying" your suppers by eating an eating regimen rich in sirtfoods staying aware of your day by day green juice.

What does the eating regimen involve?

The eating routine is executed in two stages. Stage one endures three days and limits calories to 1,000 every day, comprising of three green juices and one sirtfood-endorsed supper. Step two keeps going four days and raises day by day apportioning to 1,500 calories for every day with two green juices and two dinners.

After these stages, there is an upkeep plan that isn't centred around calories yet instead on reasonable segments, well-adjusted suppers, and topping off on fundamentally Sirt foods. The 14-day support plan highlights three dinners, one green juice, and a couple of sirtfood chomp snacks. Devotees are likewise urged to finish 30 minutes of activity five days every week-per government suggestions, yet it isn't the primary focal point of the arrangement.

The eating regimen consolidates sirtfoods and calorie limitation, the two of which may trigger the body to deliver more significant levels of sirtuins. The Sirtfood Diet book incorporates feast plans and plans to follow, yet there are a lot of other Sirtfood Diet formula books accessible.

The eating routine's makers guarantee that following the Sirtfood Diet will prompt fast weight reduction, all while keeping up bulk and shielding you from ceaseless illness. When you have finished the eating regimen, you are urged to keep, including sirtfoods and the eating routine's mark green juice into your ordinary eating routine.

Is It Effective?

The creators of the Sirtfood Diet make extreme cases, including that the eating routine can super-charge weight reduction, turn on your "thin quality" and forestall illnesses. The issue is there isn't a lot of verification to back them. Up until this point, there's no persuading proof that the Sirtfood Diet has a more significant

137

impact on weight reduction than some other calorie-confined eating routine.

What's more, albeit a large number of these nourishments have fortifying properties, there have not been any long haul human examinations to decide if eating an eating routine rich in sirtfoods has any substantial medical advantages. By the by, the Sirtfood Diet book reports the after-effects of a pilot study led by the writers and including 39 members from their wellness place. Notwithstanding, the aftereffects of this examination show up not to have been distributed anyplace else.

For multi-week, the members followed the eating regimen and practised day by day. Toward the week's end, members lost a normal of 7 pounds (3.2 kg) and kept up or even picked up the bulk. However, these outcomes are not astonishing. Confining your calorie admission to 1,000 calories and practising simultaneously will almost consistently cause weight reduction. In any case, this sort of brisk weight reduction is neither certifiable nor dependable, and this examination didn't follow members after the first week to check whether they recovered any of the weight, which is regularly the situation.

At the point when your body is vitality denied, it goes through its crisis vitality stores, or glycogen, notwithstanding consuming fat and muscle. Every atom of glycogen requires 3–4 particles of water to be put away. At the point when your body goes through glycogen, it disposes of this water also. It's known as "water weight." In the first seven day stretch of outrageous calorie limitation, just around 33% of the weight reduction originates from fat, while the other 66% originates from water, muscle and glycogen. When your calorie admission expands, your body recharges its glycogen stores, and the weight returns right.

Tragically, this kind of calorie limitation can likewise make your body bring down its metabolic rate, causing you to need considerably fewer calories every day for vitality than previously.

This eating regimen may assist you with shedding a couple of pounds before all else, yet it will probably return when the eating routine is finished. To the extent forestalling ailment, three weeks is most likely not long enough to have any quantifiable long haul sway. Then again, adding sirtfoods to your standard eating regimen over the long haul might just be a smart thought. In any case, you should avoid the eating routine and begin doing that now.

Synopsis: This eating routine may assist you with shedding pounds since it is low in calories, yet the weight is probably going to return once the eating regimen closes. The eating regimen is too short to even think about having a long haul sway on your wellbeing.

The most effective method to Follow the Sirtfood Diet:

The Sirtfood Diet has two stages that last a sum of three weeks. From that point forward, you can keep "sirtifying" your eating regimen by including, however many sirtfoods as would be prudent in your dinners. The particular plans for these two stages are found in The Sirtfood Diet book, which was composed by the eating routine's makers. You'll have to buy it to follow the eating routine. The suppers are loaded with sirtfoods however incorporate different fixings other than merely the "best 20 sirtfoods. "The more significant part of the fixings and sirtfoods are anything but difficult to discover. Be that as it may, three of the mark fixings required for these two stages —green tea powder, lovage and buckwheat — might be costly or hard to discover. A major piece of the eating routine is its green juice, which you'll have to make yourself somewhere in the range of one and multiple times every day. You will require a juicer (a blender won't work) and a kitchen scale, as the fixings are recorded by weight. The formula is beneath:

Sirtfood Green Juice

- 75 grams (2.5 Oz) kale

- **30 grams (1 Oz) arugula (rocket)**
- **5 grams parsley**
- **Two celery sticks**
- **1 cm (0.5 in) ginger**
- **a large portion of a green apple**
- **a large portion of a lemon**
- a large portion of a teaspoon matcha green tea

Squeeze all fixings aside from the green tea powder and lemon together, and empty them into a glass. Juice the lemon by hand, at that point mix both the lemon squeeze and green tea powder into your juice.

Stage One

The primary stage keeps going seven days and includes calorie limitation and loads of green juice. It is proposed to kick off your weight reduction and professed to assist you with shedding 7 pounds in seven days.

During the initial three days of stage one, calorie admission is confined to 1,000 calories. You drink three green juices for every day in addition to one feast. Every day you can look over plans in the book, which all include sirtfoods as a fundamental piece of the dinner. Feast models incorporate miso-coated tofu, the sirtfood omelette or a shrimp pan sear with buckwheat noodles. On days 4–7 of stage one, calorie admission is expanded to 1,500. This incorporates two green juices for every day and two more sirtfood-rich dinners, which you can browse the book.

Stage Two

Stage two goes on for about fourteen days. During this "support" stage, you should keep on consistently get in shape. There is no particular calorie limit for this stage. Instead, you eat three dinners brimming with sirtfoods and one green juice for every day.

After the Diet:

You may rehash these two stages as regularly as wanted for additional weight reduction. There is an assortment of Sirtfood Diet books that are loaded with plans rich in sirtfoods. You can likewise incorporate sirtfoods in your eating regimen as a bite or plans you as of now use.Right now, Sirtfood Diet turns out to be, to a higher degree, a way of life change than a one-time diet. The Sirtfood Diet comprises of two stages. Stage one keeps going seven days and consolidates calorie limitation and green juices. Step two keeps going two weeks and incorporates three dinners and one sauce.

Is Sirtfoods the New Superfoods?

There's no denying that sirtfoods are beneficial for you. They are frequently high in supplements and brimming with sound plant mixes. Also, considers have related a large number of the nourishments suggested on the Sirtfood Diet with medical advantages. For instance, eating reasonable measures of dull chocolate with a high cocoa substance may bring down the danger of coronary illness and help battle aggravation.

Drinking green tea may diminish the danger of stroke and diabetes and assist lower with blooding pressure. What's more, turmeric has mitigating properties that effect sly affect the body all in all and may even ensure against interminable, irritation related infections.

Most of the sirtfoods have exhibited medical advantages in people. In any case, proof of the medical advantages of expanding sirtuins protein levels is the starter. However, explore in creatures, and cell lines have demonstrated energizing outcomes. For instance, scientists have discovered that expanded degrees of specific sirtuin proteins lead to longer life expectancy in yeast, worms and mice.

What's more, during fasting or calorie limitation, sirtuin proteins advise the body to consume progressively fat for vitality and improve insulin affectability. One investigation in mice found that expanded sirtuin levels prompted fat misfortune. Some proof proposes that sirtuins may likewise assume a job in decreasing aggravation, hindering the advancement of tumours and easing back the improvement of coronary illness and Alzheimer's.

While considers in mice and human cell lines have demonstrated positive outcomes, there have been no human investigations looking at the impacts of expanding sirtuin levels. Along these lines, in the case of developing sirtuin protein levels in the body will prompt longer life expectancy or a lower danger of malignant growth in people is obscure.

What would you be able to eat on the Sirtfood Diet?

The Sirtfood Diet feature grabbers are red wine, and dim chocolate since the two of them happen to be high in sirtuin activators. Even though that is not the entire picture and you won't feel the impacts by mainlining Merlot and Green and Blacks (more's the pity).

The Sirtfood Diet plan centres around increasing your admission of sound sirtfoods. These incorporate the accompanying: apples, organic citrus products, parsley, escapades, blueberries, green tea, soy, strawberries, turmeric, red onion, rocket and that old wellbeing darling's preferred kale.

Strikingly, another top sirtfood is espresso, which is welcome news in case you're exhausted of being advised to remove caffeine. Nations, where individuals as of now expend an immense number of sirtfoods, incorporate Japan and Italy, which are both routinely positioned among the world's most advantageous nations.

Is there a Sirtfood Diet plan?

Truly there is! For the first week, you limit your admission to 1000 calories every day, which incorporates devouring three sirtfood green juices and one sirtfood lavish supper daily. The next week you up to your access to 1500 calories every day and eat two sirtfood-rich dinners and two green juices. Be that as it may, in the long haul there is no set arrangement, it's everything about modifying your way of life to incorporate whatever number sirtfoods as could reasonably be expected, which should cause you to feel more advantageous and increasingly fiery.

Who concocted the Sirtfood Diet?

A couple of creators and wellbeing specialists called Aidan Goggins and Glen Matten, whose spotlight has consistently been on proper dieting instead of weight reduction. In the book The Sirtfood Diet, the pair spread out a dinner plan which includes drinking three sirtfood green squeezes a day joined by adjusted sirtfood-rich suppers, for example, 'buckwheat and prawn pan sear' or 'smoked salmon sirt super salad.'

Synopsis:

The Sirtfood Diet depends on to inquire about on sirtuins, a gathering of proteins that direct a few capacities in the body. Certain nourishments called sirtfoods may make the body produce a higher amount of these proteins. The vast majority of the sirtfoods have displayed restorative points of interest in individuals. Regardless, evidence of the medicinal points of interest of extending sirtuins protein levels is the starter.

Chapter 2: How Do Sirtfood Diet Works?

You may have known about the Sirtfood Plan previously - mainly since it was accounted for vocalist Adele lost 50lbs after the arrangement - however, do you know what it is? The eating plan characterizes the 20 nourishments that turn on your alleged 'thin qualities', boosting your digestion and your vitality levels. It stipulates that you could lose 7lbs in 7 days. The eating plan will change how you do proper dieting. It might seem like a non-easy to use the name. However, it's one you'll be catching wind of a great deal. Since the 'Sirt' in Sirtfoods is shorthand for the sirtuin qualities, a gathering of classes nicknamed the 'thin qualities' that work, in all honesty, similar to enchantment.

Eating these nourishments, state the makers of the arrangement, nutritionists Aidan Goggins and Glen Matten, turns on these qualities and "mirrors the impacts of calorie limitation, fasting and exercise". It initiates a reusing procedure in the body, "that gets out the cell garbage and mess which aggregates after some time and causes sick wellbeing and loss of essentialness," compose the creators.

What are Sirtuins?

Sirtuins are a group of proteins that manage cell wellbeing. Sirtuins assume a crucial job in controlling cell homeostasis. Homeostasis includes keeping the cell in balance. Protein may seem like dietary protein — what's found in beans and meats and well, protein shakes — however right now discussing atoms called proteins, which work all through the body's phones in various capacities. Consider proteins the divisions at an organization, everyone concentrating without anyone else specific ability while planning with different offices.

A notable protein in the body is haemoglobin, which is a piece of the globin group of proteins and is liable for shipping oxygen all through your blood. The myoglobin is the haemoglobin's partner, and together they make up the globin family. Your body has almost 60,000 groups of proteins — a lot of offices! — and sirtuins are one of those families. While haemoglobin is one of every a group of two proteins, sirtuins are a group of seven.

Of the seven sirtuins in the cell, three of them work in the mitochondria, three of them work in the core, and one of them works in the cytoplasm, each assuming an assortment of jobs. The first job of sirtuins, notwithstanding, is that they expel acetyl bunches from different proteins.

Acetyl bunches control explicit responses. They're physical labels on proteins that different proteins perceive will respond with them. If proteins are the branches of the cell and DNA is the CEO, the acetyl bunches are the accessibility status of every office head. For instance, if a protein is accessible, at that point, the sirtuin can work with it to get something going, similarly as the CEO can work with an available division head to get something going.

One way that sirtuins work is by expelling acetyl gatherings (de acetylating) organic proteins, for example, histones. For instance, sirtuins deacetylate histones, proteins that are a piece of a dense type of DNA called chromatin. The histone is a substantial massive protein that the DNA folds itself over. Consider it a Christmas tree, and the DNA strand is the strand of lights. At the point when the histones have an acetyl gathering, the chromatin is open or loosened up.

This loosened up chromatin implies the DNA is being deciphered, a necessary procedure. However, it doesn't have to remain loosened up, as it's helpless against harm right now, similar to the Christmas lights could get tangled or the bulbs can get harmed when they're clumsy or up for a long time. At the point when sirtuins deacetylate the histones, the chromatin is shut, or firmly and perfectly twisted, which means quality articulation is halted or quieted.

We've just thought about sirtuins for around 20 years, and their essential capacity was found during the 1990s. From that point forward, analysts have run to contemplate them, distinguishing their significance while likewise bringing up issues about what else we can find out about them.

How Sirtuins Regulate Cellular Health with NAD+

Think about your body's cells like an office. In the workplace, numerous individuals are chipping away at different undertakings with an ultimate objective: remain beneficial and effectively satisfy the strategic the organization for whatever length of time that conceivable. In the cells, numerous pieces are taking a shot at different errands with an ultimate objective, as well: remain sound and capacity productively for whatever length of time that conceivable. Similarly, as needs in the organization change, because of different inward and outer variables, so do requirements in the cells. Somebody needs to run the workplace, controlling what completes when, who will do it and when to switch course. In the workplace, that would be your CEO.

On the off chance that sirtuins are an organization's CEO, at that point, NAD+ is the cash that pays the pay of the CEO and representatives, all while keeping the lights on and the workplace space lease paid. An organization, and the body, can't work without it. Be that as it may, levels of NAD+ decrease with age, restricting the capacity of sirtuins with age also. Like everything in the human body, it isn't so necessary. Sirtuins oversee everything that occurs in your cells.

Synopsis:

Sirtuins are a group of proteins that assume a job in cell wellbeing.NAD+ is indispensable to cell digestion and many other natural procedures. Sirtuins work with acetyl bunches by doing what's called deacetylation. This implies they perceive there's an acetyl bunch on an atom at that point evacuate the acetyl gathering, which tees up the particle for its activity.

Chapter 3: Benefits Of Sirtfood Diet

Here are three motivations to take a pass on the sirtfood food:

1. The sirtfood diet estimates achievement just regarding weight reduction.

I've said it previously, and I'll state it once more: Weight is a determinant of wellbeing. However, it's not alone. To gauge somebody's wellbeing accomplishment on whether they lose X pounds in X measure of time disregards the various advantages of nourishment. It additionally has supplements that can advance a few substantial capacities and is regularly a euphoric encounter established in the convention. For by and broad wellbeing, there's quite a lot more to concentrate on than fundamentally appearance, and estimating achievement just regarding weight reduction is incomprehensible.

2. It's prohibitive, which can harm your association with nourishment.

This eating routine underlines an admission of 1,000 to 1,500 calories for every day, which is a lot of lower than the vast majority need. At the point when we severely limit our nourishment consumption, our natural response is to gorge. Your body is keen, and it thinks about this absence of sustenance as an assault. Along these lines, we will in general overcompensate, which is the reason we as a whole can identify with being "hangry" and therefore overindulging whenever we're at last allowed to eat. Rehearsing careful and natural eating is a more supportable course than confining nourishment.

3. The sirtfood diet isn't science-based.

While there is some questionable research about the advantages of sirtuins, there's practically zero research about the particular sirtfood diet. Additionally, we as of now have a few rules set up that have been altogether looked into and tried for quite a long time. In case you're lost on what "solid nourishment" is, this is a superior spot to begin.

It's beautiful if you need to consolidate a couple of sirtfoods into an eating plan. Nourishments like green tea, organic product, dim chocolate, and kale all include a spot inside a smart dieting design! In any case, holding fast to a program with such exacting pass-or-bomb prerequisites is unreasonable and could be destructive to your association with nourishment. By consolidating an eating plan that is loaded with assortment and eating carefully, you'll have the option to set up a long haul, maintainable association with nourishment. Cheers to that!

What are the advantages?

You will get more fit on the off chance that you follow this eating regimen intently. "Regardless of whether you're eating 1,000 calories of tacos, 1,000 calories of kale, or 1,000 calories of snickerdoodles, you will get more fit at 1,000 calories!" says Dr Youdim. In any case, she additionally brings up that you can have accomplishment with a progressively sensible calorie limitation. The run of the mill every day caloric admission of somebody not on an eating routine is 2,000 to 2,200, so decreasing to 1,500 is as yet confining and would be a successful weight reduction procedure for most, she says.

Are there any safety measures?

This arrangement is severe with little squirm room or substitutions, and weight reduction must be kept up if the low caloric admission is likewise kept up, making it hard to hold fast to the long haul. That implies any weight you lost in the initial seven days is probably going to be recovered after you finish, says Dr Youdin. Her primary concern? "Constraining protein admission with juices will bring about lost bulk. Losing muscle is synonymous with dropping your metabolic rate or 'digestion,' making weight upkeep increasingly troublesome," she says.

What do practical nourishment specialists need to state about it?

Generally speaking, master input on the Sirtfood Diet is blended. The uplifting news: The eating regimen seems to be stacked with sound nourishments. "There is broad research that features the numerous advantages of a portion of the nourishments got down on about this eating routine, similar to espresso, green tea, dull chocolate, and dim verdant greens," says Jessica Cording, R.D., enrolled dietitian and wellbeing mentor.

Vast numbers of these nourishments may likewise bolster substantial weight reduction, says Frances Large man-Roth, R.D., however, whether they advance weight reduction by actuating sirtuins stays to be demonstrated. "The nourishments advanced on the eating routine are ones that battle aggravation and would be valuable for anybody to add to their eating regimen yet not because they help sirtuins," she says. "Because nourishment contains a specific supplement connected to digestion doesn't imply that nourishment causes programmed weight reduction— it is doubtful to turn on a 'thin quality' with nourishment."Moreover, while these "sirtfoods" are without a doubt substantial, Large man-Roth says somebody would need to ensure they're additionally balancing their suppers with sound fats and proteins.

Concerning the structure of the eating routine, it may not be significant. However, Cording figures it could be an agreeable choice for individuals who are keen on a weight-reduction plan that has some structure and offers space for adaptability and customization. "I welcome that it's a 'diet of incorporation' versus one concentrated basically on limiting nourishments," she says. So, Cording concedes that the juice-substantial beginning piece of Phase One is a bit lower in calories than what she'd regularly prescribe. Yet, the later stages, which incorporate a more unhealthy objective and healthy nourishment, are, to some degree, increasingly economical.

Synopsis:

Nourishment is loaded with vitality, which permits you to do things like showering, practising and relaxing. The sirtfood diet depends on the possibility that specific nourishments actuate sirtuins in your body, which are explicit proteins speculated to receive different rewards, from shielding cells in your body from aggravation to turning around maturing

Chapter 4: Best Sirt Diet Foods

The rundown of the "best 20 sirtfoods" gave by the Sirtfood Diet incorporates:

- Kale
- **Red wine**
- **Strawberries**
- **Onions**
- **Soy**
- **Parsley**
- **Additional virgin olive oil**
- **Dim chocolate (85% cocoa)**
- **Matcha green tea**
- **Buckwheat**
- **Turmeric**
- **Pecans**
- **Arugula (rocket)**
- **Superior stew**
- **Lovage**
- **Medjool dates**
- **Red chicory**
- Blueberries

Kale as Diet Food

Kale is a green, verdant, cruciferous vegetable that is wealthy in supplements. It might offer a scope of medical advantages for the entire body. It is an individual from the mustard or Brassicaceae, family, as are cabbage and Brussels grows. Potential advantages incorporate overseeing circulatory strain, boosting stomach related wellbeing, and ensuring against malignant growth and type 2 diabetes.

Advantages

Devouring kale may help support stomach related wellbeing, among different benefits. Kale contains fibre, cancer prevention agents, calcium, nutrients C and K, iron, and a full scope of different supplements that can help forestall various medical issues.

Cancer prevention agents help the body expel undesirable poisons that outcome from diagnostic procedures and ecological weights. These poisons, known as free radicals, are unsteady particles. On the off chance that too many developers in the body, they can prompt cell harm. This may bring about medical issues, for example, irritation and ailments. Specialists accept that free radicals may assume a job in the advancement of the disease, for instance.

Diabetes

The American Diabetes Association suggest devouring nourishments that are plentiful in nutrients, minerals, fibre, and cancer prevention agents. There is proof that a portion of these may offer security against diabetes.

Fibre: A recent report presumed that individuals who devour the most elevated measures of dietary fibre seem to have a lower danger of creating type 2 diabetes. Eating dietary fibre may likewise bring down blood glucose levels, the creators note.

Cell reinforcements: Authors of a 2012 article note that high glucose levels can trigger the generation of free radicals. They note that cancer prevention agents, for example, nutrient C and alpha-linolenic corrosive (ALA), can help lessen entanglements that may happen with diabetes. Both of these cancer prevention agents are available in kale.

Coronary illness

Different supplements in kale may bolster heart wellbeing.

Potassium: The American Heart Association (AHA) prescribe expanding the admission of potassium while decreasing the utilization of included salt, or sodium. This, state the AHA, can diminish the danger of hypertension and cardiovascular sickness. A cup of cooked kale gives 3.6% of a grown-up's everyday requirements for potassium.

Fibre: A Cochrane survey from 2016 found a connection between expending fibre and a lower blood lipid (fat) levels and circulatory strain. Individuals who consumed more fibre were bound to have lower levels of total cholesterol and low-thickness lipoprotein (LDL) or "awful" cholesterol. Individuals need both dissolvable and insoluble fibre.

Kale and green vegetables that contain chlorophyll can help keep the body from engrossing heterocyclic amines. These synthetic compounds happen when individuals flame broil creature determined nourishments at a high temperature. Specialists have connected them with malignancy.

The human body can't assimilate a lot of chlorophyll; however, chlorophyll ties to these cancer-causing agents and keeps the body from retaining them. Right now, it may restrict the danger of malignant growth, and blending a chargrilled steak with green vegetables may help lessen the adverse effect.

Cell reinforcements: Nutrient C, beta carotene, selenium, and different cell reinforcements in kale may help forestall disease. Studies have not discovered that enhancements have a similar impact. Yet, individuals who have a high admission of foods grown from the ground seem to have a lower danger of creating different tumours. This might be because of the cell reinforcements these nourishments contain.

Fibre: A high utilization of fibre may help decrease the danger of colorectal disease, as indicated by an investigation from 2015.

Bone wellbeing

Calcium and phosphorus are pivotal for sound bone development. Some examination has recommended that a high admission of nutrient K may help decrease the danger of bone cracks. A cup of cooked kale gives just about multiple times a grown-up's daily requirement for nutrient K, around 18% of their calcium need, and about 7% of the day by day phosphorus necessity.

Absorption

Kale is high in fibre and water, the two of which help forestall obstruction and advance normality and a stable stomach related tract.

Skin and hair

Kale is a decent wellspring of beta-carotene, the carotenoid that the body changes over into nutrient An as it needs it. Beta-carotene and nutrient An are essential for the development and support of all body tissues, including the skin and hair. The body utilizes nutrient C to fabricate and look after collagen, a protein that gives structure to skin, hair, and bones. Nutrient C is likewise present in kale. A cup of cooked kale offers at any rate 20% of an individual's day by day requirement for nutrient An and over 23% of the day by day necessity for nutrient C.

Eye wellbeing

Kale contains lutein and zeaxanthin, a cell reinforcement blend that may help decrease the danger of old enough related macular degeneration. Nutrient C, nutrient E, beta-carotene, and zinc additionally assume a job in eye wellbeing. These are available in kale.

Red Wine as Diet food

Research shows that resveratrol, a fixing found in grapes, berries and red wine can help transform fat into calorie-consuming 'dark-coloured' fat. Simply drink capably! ... They found that in spite of a high-fat eating routine, the mice put on 40% less weight than creatures not bolstered the compound.

Wine darlings celebrate! Research has demonstrated that fixing in grapes, berries and red wine can transform abundance fat into calorie-consuming "dark coloured" fat. The revelation proposes that diets containing the substance, resveratrol, may help battle weight.

Researchers gave mice measures of resveratrol identical to people devouring 12 ounces of organic product every day. They found that in spite of a high-fat eating regimen, the mice put on 40% less weight than creatures not bolstered the compound.

Starting to eat better used to mean removing every "awful" nourishment and beverages to get in shape, and liquor was commonly the first to go. In addition to the fact that it adds additional calories, yet it likewise makes it simpler to store carbs as fat as opposed to consuming them off. Be that as it may, for some, individuals, adhering to an eating plan that restricts alcohol isn't just unsavoury and troublesome, yet additionally probably not going to be feasible for long haul objectives.

Luckily, counting calories presently can mean numerous things, from restricting the utilization of incendiary nourishments to removing gluten to embracing the eating examples of a particular locale. Furthermore, it's about something beyond dropping pounds: Maintaining heart wellbeing, boosting your resistant framework, amending a wellbeing condition or essentially holding dietary patterns under wraps are generally regular purposes behind after an eating plan.

Research has demonstrated that, regardless of whether you are slimming down to shed pounds, you don't need to overlook wine from your way of life. A portion of the present most famous eating regimens permits (and, sometimes, support!) moderate wine utilization.

Not all wine darlings are made the equivalent, which means various weight control plans will have multiple impacts on everybody. Considering your way of life inclinations, and counselling with your primary care physician about your wellbeing and wellbeing related decisions will enable you to pick what's appropriate for you.

Here are mainstream, wine-accommodating eating plans that you've presumably known about, with information and guidance from specialists in the wellbeing and health field.

Mediterranean eating routine

A most loved among wine consumers, the Mediterranean eating routine copies the eating examples of individuals local to territories that fringe the Mediterranean Sea, for example, Italy, Greece, southern France and Spain. Portrayed by natural products, vegetables, fish, nuts, entire grains, olive oil and moderate wine utilization, the eating routine has been appeared to have various advantages, including better liver wellbeing and lower weight gain.

Moderate wine utilization was remembered for this eating regimen principally because it's a piece of the general propensities for individuals who live on the Mediterranean. Yet, wine's science-sponsored potential medical advantages are the reason it remains some portion of the arrangement.

"On the Mediterranean eating routine, you can have a wine [because the eating regimen is] low on carbs, and it's low on fat, so when you're drinking liquor, it won't influence you to such an extent."

However, the eating routine is entirely remiss on rules, visit wine consumers despite everything should be aware of what they're expending. "As of late, I had a customer who's an authority of wine—he had like 800 jugs in his loft—and he resembles, 'I drink [frequently]. On a Thursday night, my better half and I will part a jug of wine,'" Rissetto said. "So I needed to truly concentrate on reducing the starch heap of his every day admission with the goal that he could get in shape and still beverage wine."

The DASH (Dietary Approaches to Stop Hypertension) diet is a nearby cousin of the Mediterranean eating routine, made considering circulatory strain. It stresses organic products, vegetables, entire grains and low-fat dairy items while restricting fats.

In contrast to the Mediterranean eating routine, DASH neither endorses nor disallows liquor utilization. Yet, the MIND (Mediterranean-DASH diet Intervention for Neurodegenerative Delay) diet, a mixture of the Mediterranean and DASH eat fewer carbs that were created by specialists who trust it can decrease psychological decay as individuals age, includes wine.

Mitigating diet

What separates this eating regimen is the explanation the vast majority are on it: Inflammation can show in the body in various ways, including joint pain, asthma, coronary illness, weight gain, gut issues, skin issues and that's only the tip of the iceberg. Holding fast to a calming diet can help with one or a blend of these issues.

Like the Mediterranean eating routine, there is no rundown of explicit nourishments that you can or can't eat on a calming diet; it's all the more a guide for the sorts of things you can devour. Mitigating nourishments that are energized incorporate verdant greens, healthy fats, for example, fish and nuts, and wine with some restraint.

Need to get familiar with how wine can be a piece of a sound way of life? Pursue Wine Spectator's free Wine and Healthy Living email pamphlet and get the most recent wellbeing news, feel-great plans, health tips and more conveyed directly to your inbox each other week!

Red wine is explicitly viewed as a feature of this eating routine since it usually contains mitigating polyphenols, for example, resveratrol. "The cell reinforcement properties in red wine can help forestall free extreme harm, which is a contributory factor in advancing aggravation the body," said Tracy Lockwood Beckerman, an enrolled dietitian in New York City and originator of the organization Tracy Nutrition.

In any case, she brings up, while contemplates have been done on resveratrol as an enhancement to help with issues, for example, joint agony and diabetes, there is no proof yet that the measure of resveratrol found in one glass of wine would be sufficient to affect—and drinking past prescribed breaking points to get those medical advantages is profoundly ill-advised. It's smarter to adhere to a balanced eating regimen of mitigating nourishment and refreshments.

Sans gluten diet

"This is an eating regimen principally for patients who have celiac [disease], or gluten affectability," Dr Bindiya Gandhi, a Georgia-based doctor, disclosed to Wine Spectator. "I will likewise prescribe this eating routine to patients with irritation, PCOS [Polycystic Ovary Syndrome] and immune system issues."

The name should warn you to the way that on this eating routine, you should dodge gluten, a protein found in wheat, rye, grain and some different grains. You can have as a lot of wine as you need (however we despite everything prescribe drinking with some restraint for your general wellbeing).

In any case, while wine, by and large, is viewed as sans gluten, the individuals who are particularly touchy to gluten should give close consideration to precisely how their wine is made. Gluten can at times be fixing in some fining operators or wine-barrel sealants. And still, after all that, however, gluten levels likely wouldn't be sufficiently high to enrol in your body.

Strawberry as diet food

The energizing examination that is being done shows that the unique healthful segments in strawberries may have the option to invigorate your digestion and help smother your craving. They can control glucose and can likewise assist you with getting in shape.

It is no big surprise that researchers over the United States, in Sweden and different nations have been inquiring about the miracles of the strawberry and finding more proof of its medical advantages. There is no uncertainty that strawberries have joined the other demigods of overly nutritious natural product, for example, blueberries, fruits, cranberries and pomegranates.

What Gives Strawberries Their Nutritional Punch?

Strawberries are solid nourishment to eat to shed pounds because there are 49 calories in a single cup of berries. They are additionally stacked with Vitamin C, 3 grams of fibre, and some calcium, magnesium, and potassium.

Strawberries are rich wellsprings of phenolic cancer prevention agents that can help:

- turn around irritation
- **help in weight reduction**
- decrease the danger of ceaseless sickness.

College of Illinois scientists found that the most bounteous cancer prevention agents in strawberries are elegiac corrosive, just as the flavonoids quercetin, kaempferol anthocyanin and catechin. They further brought up that strawberry removes have appeared to restrain COX catalysts in research centre investigations. This would imply that strawberries could help decrease aggravation and agony.

Research on Strawberries and Disease

Research results demonstrate that strawberries can offer wholesome help to battle maturing and sickness. In vitro research centre examinations from Cornell University propose that strawberry concentrates may help repress the development of liver disease cells. Concentrates with research facility creatures showed advantages of strawberries for the maturing

161

cerebrum. Writing in the Journal of Medicinal Food researchers from Clemson University inspected the disease battling capability of different berries. They note: "Plants are demonstrated wellsprings of the valuable enemy of a tumour and chemopreventative mixes. Subsequently, recognizable proof of phytochemicals helpful in dietary anticipation and intercession of malignant growth is of central significance.

Strawberries Help Protect the Heart

Strawberry has direct calming impacts, restraining the actuation of qualities and compounds that advance irritation. A large portion of this advantage is because of another gathering of phenolic cell reinforcements called anthocyanins, which help give ready strawberries their rich red shading. Anthocyanins decline the danger of coronary illness and stroke by shielding veins from the impacts of mileage.

Strawberries Promote Weight Loss

The ellagic corrosive and anthocyaninsfound in fruits help weight reduction in any event three different ways:

1) Constant aggravation obstructs the hormones engaged with keeping you lean. 2) Calming nourishments like strawberries help reestablish typical capacity to weight-decreasing hormones.

3) Anthocyanins increment the body's creation of a hormone called adiponectin, which animates your digestion and smothers your hunger.

Both elegiac corrosive and anthocyanins moderate the pace of assimilation of bland nourishments, controlling the ascent in glucose that follows a boring dinner. This impact is utilized to control glucose in individuals with grown-up beginning (Type 2) diabetes.

Natural Strawberries Have More Nutrition

I prescribe naturally developed strawberries. Natural strawberries have been appeared to have more elevated levels of nutrient C and than expectedly grown berries, because of a higher substance of phenolic cell reinforcements. In an intriguing report, analysts from Washington State University contrasted natural strawberries and ranches with traditional fruits and homesteads. They saw the natural fruits as higher in quality, and the dirt to be more beneficial. In particular, in contrast with the routinely developed berries, the natural strawberries had more top all out cancer prevention agents, ascorbic corrosive, and complete phenolic.

Appreciating Strawberries

Strawberries give you a flavour, shading, and fragrance, arousing your taste buds to the crisp, characteristic nourishments your body should be reliable and fundamental. When looking for berries, freshness is significant. Distinguish strawberries that are brilliant red and firm. Fruits are an extraordinary bite of pastry and add shading and flavour to solid plans. Ordinarily sweet and delicious, strawberries are a great delight and make a remarkable sound treat.

Include a bunch of cut strawberries to:

- Grain or granola
- **Hot oats**
- **Smoothies**
- Yoghurt

You can eat new or solidified strawberries as a tidbit or sweet whenever.

Onion as diet food:

"Onions are super-sound," said Victoria Jarzabkowski, a nutritionist with the Fitness Institute of Texas at the University of Texas at Austin. "They are magnificent wellsprings of nutrient C, sulphuric mixes, flavonoids and phytochemicals."

Flavonoids are answerable for colours in many foods grown from the ground. Studies have indicated that they may help diminish the danger of Parkinson's infection, cardiovascular sickness and stroke.

An unusually significant flavonoid in onions is quercetin, which goes about as a cell reinforcement that might be connected to forestalling disease. "It likewise may have heart medical advantages. However, more examinations should be done," said Angela Lemond.

Quercetin has a large group of different advantages, also, as per the University of Maryland Medical Center, diminishing the side effects of bladder diseases, advancing prostate wellbeing and bringing down pulse. Other significant phytochemicals in onions are disulfides, trisulfides, cepaene and vinyldithiins. They all are useful in keeping up great wellbeing and have anticancer and antimicrobial properties, as per the National Onion Association.

Somewhat on account of their utilization in cooking the world over, onions are among the most critical wellsprings of cancer prevention agents in the human eating routine, as per a 2002 report in the diary Phytotherapy Research. Their elevated levels of cell reinforcements give onions their unmistakable sweetness and smell."Cell reinforcements help forestall harm and malignant growth. Amino acids are the essential structure hinder for protein, and protein is utilized in for all intents and purposes each vital capacity in the body."

Sulfides in onions contain essential amino acids. "Sulfur is one of the most widely recognized minerals in our body that helps with protein union and working of cell structures," said Lemond.

"I like to suggest eating onions since they include season without salt and sugar," Jarzabkowski said. Onions are low in calories (45 for every serving), low in sodium, and contain no fat or cholesterol. Moreover, onions contain fibre and folic corrosive, a B nutrient that enables the body to make solid new cells. Onions are sound whether they're crude or cooked. However, coarse onions have more elevated levels of natural sulfur intensifies that give numerous advantages, as indicated by the BBC. A recent report in the Journal of Agricultural and Food Chemistry found that there is a high centralization of flavonoids in the external layers of onion tissue, so you'll need to be mindful to evacuate as meagre of the consumable piece of the onion as conceivable when stripping it. Here are the nourishment realities for onions, as per the U.S. Nourishment and Drug

165

Administration, which controls nourishment naming through the National Labeling and Education Act.

Nourishment realities

Serving size: 1 medium onionCalories: 45 (Calories from Fat: 0)

Sum per servingPercent Daily Values (%DV) depend on a 2,000-calorie diet.

Absolute fat: 0g (0%)

Absolute Carbohydrate: 11gDietary Fiber 3g (12%) Sugars 9g

Cholesterol: 0mg (0%) Sodium: 5mg (0%) Potassium: 190mg (5%) Protein: 1g

Nutrient A: (0%) Vitamin C: (20%) Calcium: (4%) Iron: (4%)

Medical advantages :

Heart wellbeing

As per Jarzabkowski, onions energize a solid heart from multiple points of view, including "bringing down pulse and bringing down cardiovascular failure hazard." A recent report in the diary Thrombosis Research recommended that sulfur goes about as characteristic blood more slender and forestalls blood platelets from amassing. At the point when platelets bunch, the hazard for coronary failure or stroke increments. This examination further backings a comparable 1992 investigation in Thrombosis Research that concentrated on sulfurs in garlic. Moreover, a 1987 creature study in the Journal of Hypertension exhibited deferred or decreased beginning of hypertension with sulfur admission. In any case, the creators said more research was expected to decide whether this advantage may be found in people.

As of late, wellbeing specialists have seen a connection between informing atoms called oxylipins and elevated cholesterol the board. A recent report in the diary Redox Biology found that expending onions increments oxylipins that help control blood fat levels and levels of cholesterol.

The quercetin in onions may likewise help forestall plaque development in the supply routes, which diminishes the danger of coronary failure and stroke, as per the University of Maryland Medical Center. Be that as it may, since a large portion of the investigations right now centred around creatures, more research is expected to comprehend the impacts in people.

Soy as Diet food:

Soy items originate from soybeans. Soybeans are vegetables that have been a piece of Asian eating regimens for a considerable length of time. Soybeans are utilized to make tofu, soymilk, soy flour, miso and numerous different nourishments. In contrast to other plant nourishments, soybeans have a high protein content, identical to creature food sources. Like meat, soy is a complete protein. This implies it gives all the essential amino acids that your body needs yet can't create without anyone else. In addition to the fact that soy is a decent wellspring of protein, it additionally gives numerous other useful supplements. Soy contains two sound sorts of fat, called omega-3 and omega-6 unsaturated fats. Soy is likewise a fantastic wellspring of folate, iron, calcium, nutrient D, zinc, insoluble fibre, phosphorus, copper, magnesium, manganese and B nutrients.

Soy has numerous medical advantages. It has been connected to decreasing menopausal side effects, for example, night sweats and hot flashes. Soy can expand bone thickness, along these lines offering insurance against osteoporosis. Soy can likewise assist lower with blooding cholesterol levels, helping with diminishing the danger of coronary illness.

Nourishment that contains soy

- Tofu
- **Soy drinks**
- **Soy milk**

- **Green soybeans**
- **Broiled soy nuts**
- **Soy flour**
- **Soy protein powder**
- **Veggie sausages or burgers**
- **"Meatless" lunch meats**
- Potential wellbeing concern

Soy contains such flavones, which are original mixes with estrogen-like properties. There is information to recommend that along these lines; soy can effect sly affect estrogen-subordinate bosom malignancy. If you are concerned, address your PCP.

A few people are hypersensitive to soy.

Eating and cooking with soy

Figuring out how to utilize and cook with soy items may appear to be troublesome from the start. Even though soy may appear to be new, it is found in numerous nourishments that are as of now generally expended. For instance, soybean oil is a fixing in like manner nourishments, for example, mayonnaise, margarine and plate of mixed greens dressing.

Tofu

Tofu is made generally from cooked soybeans. Tofu arrives in an assortment of surfaces and flavours. There are two general classifications of tofu: firm and delicate (smooth). Firm sorts of tofu have more soy protein than the milder assortments. Either structure can be prepared, cooked, flame-broiled, seared or eaten crude. Tofu can be eaten entire, squashed, cubed or consolidated in an assortment of delicious blends to make a large number of nutritious and delightful dishes.

Soymilk

Soymilk is produced using ground soybeans blended in with water to deliver a milk-like fluid. It very well may be utilized rather than milk for youngsters beyond two years old and grown-ups. Soymilk is incredible with grain and can likewise be used when cooking. Soymilk, for the most part, comes plain or in an assortment of flavours, for example, vanilla, chocolate and espresso. Search for soy drinks that are improved with calcium and nutrient D.

Soy nuts

Cooked soy nuts are not so many nuts. They are entire soybeans that have been absorbed water and afterwards prepared to a brilliant dark-coloured. Soy nuts arrive in an assortment of delicious flavours and are comparative in surface and taste to peanuts. You can discover a variety of delicious simmered soy nuts in wellbeing or forte nourishment stores and numerous supermarkets.

Tempeh

Tempeh is produced using entire, cooked soybeans that are framed into a chewy soybean cake. It tends to be marinated and added to a large number of your preferred dishes. It is regularly utilized as a meat substitute and assumes the kind of different fixings it is being cooked with. Tempeh is usually cut and seared until its surface is brilliant darker. Tempeh is found in the solidified nourishment area and remains new in the cooler for a long time.

What amount of soy?

There is right now no proposal on how much soy you ought to devour every day. Be that as it may, soy items ought to be a piece of a stable, well-adjusted eating routine. By and large, assortment and control are vital to proper dieting.

Bring soy gradually into your eating regimen by including modest quantities every day or blending it in with nourishments you as of now eat and appreciate. As you become acclimated to the taste and surface of the different soy items, continue including more. The excellence of some soy items is that they have a gentle or nonpartisan flavour, which makes them simple to consolidate into dishes.

The accompanying servings are identical to one serving of soy as indicated by Canada's Food Guide to Healthy Eating:

- 1/3 cup tofu (any surface)
- **1 cup braced soy drink**
- **1.5 ounces (50g) soy cheddar**
- 3/4 cup soy yoghurt

Approaches to remember more soy for your eating regimen

There are numerous straightforward approaches to fuse soy into your eating regimen. Follow Canada's Food Guide to Healthy diet as a beginning stage.

In the Grain Products nutritional category:

- use soy flour rather than a generally useful meal in preparing plans
- **to appreciate soy cornmeal rather than cereal**
- pick a soy grain

In the Vegetables and Fruit nutritional category:

- include soybeans (cooked or canned) or soy nuts to your plate of mixed greens.
- **Appreciate steamed edamame (green soybeans) as a sound tidbit or added to pan sear. They are accessible in the solidified nourishments area of most supermarkets.**
- Mix delicate (smooth) tofu or soy yoghurt with a natural product, squeeze and ice 3D squares in a blender for a marvellous breakfast shake.

In the Milk Products nutrition type:

- incorporate soy refreshments advanced with calcium and nutrient D
- **utilize invigorated soy refreshments in your espresso or on your oat**
- **supplant the cream in sweets with soymilk or soy yoghurt**
- **search for soy forms of frozen yoghurt and yoghurts.**
- soy cheeses work extraordinary in pasta and pizza plans

In the Meat and Alternatives nutrition class:

- incorporate protein-rich tofu rather than ground hamburger in tacos, bean stew or spaghetti sauce.
- **Block firm tofu and add to pan sear. Dark-coloured it in sesame oil and add to your veggies.**
- **Attempt a soy-based burger or veggie burger.**
- **Attempt the delectable and helpful soy items accessible that are made to possess a flavour like ham, pepperoni, bologna and prepared to-eat hotdog.**
- Include pureed tofu or ground soy hotdog to your next meatloaf.

Parsley as diet food:

Parsley, which has the logical name Petroselinum crissum, is a type of Petroselinum, an individual from the group of Apiaceous plants. Different plants in the Apiaceous family incorporate carrots, celery and various herbs, similar to cumin, dill and anise.

It is initially local to the focal Mediterranean district, where even today it's as yet the feature of a considerable lot of the zone's territorial plans. Parsley herb and essential oil have been utilized as normal detox cures, diuretics, and clean and mitigating specialists for a considerable length of time in society drug. Nations and areas, for example, southern Italy, Algeria and Tunisia were a portion of the principal producers of this mending herb. The fantastic medical advantages of this herb come using its dynamic fixings, which studies show include:

- phenolic mixes
- **cancer prevention agent flavonoids**
- **carotenoids**
- **ascorbic corrosive**
- **fundamental oils like myristicin and apiol**
- different supplements like nutrients K, C and A

As indicated by a 2013 report in the Journal of Traditional Chinese Medicine, parsley has been utilized as "treatment of the gastrointestinal issue, hypertension, heart illness, urinary malady, diabetes and different dermal ailments in customary and old stories drugs."

Types

There are two fundamental sorts of parsley plants utilized as herbs in plans:

- Wavy leaf parsley, likewise called French parsley
- Italian, or level leaf parsley

Flat-leaf Italian parsley is all the more firmly identified with the wild parsley species that was first developed in the Mediterranean. Be that as it may, a few people incline toward the wavy leaf assortment due to its enlivening appearance when it's utilized over plans. The two kinds taste fundamentally the same as somebody who isn't incredibly acquainted with them, and both offer comparable medical advantages. Even though it's not seen particularly in the U.S., there is another kind of parsley: Hamburg root parsley, which seems to be like its relative the parsnip. This root vegetable plant is developed and utilized in parts of the world like the Middle East. Root parsley is likewise utilized in some European foods, where it's additional to dishes like soups and stews, or eaten crude.

Goes about as Natural Diuretic and Helps Relieve Bloating

Solid proof exists that parsley can be utilized as a characteristic diuretic to help diminish water maintenance and simplicity swelling, as per a 2002 survey done at the American University of Beirut.

In the examination, rodents given parsley seed extricate demonstrated a considerable increment in the volume of pee they created over the 24 hours following. Parsley benefits stomach related wellbeing since it invigorates kidney generation of pee and draws abundance water out of the mid-region, where it can cause inconvenience and acid reflux.

Improves Digestion and Kidney Health

Parsley and its organic oil are utilized to treat various gastrointestinal manifestations and clutters, including gas, stoppage, swelling, acid reflux and queasiness.

As per Ayurveda rehearses, parsley benefits assimilation because the organic oil can help increment bile generation and useful gastric juices that are required for legitimate protein capacities engaged with nourishment and supplement ingestion. The oil can be added to a shower or weakened and scoured on the stomach region for alleviation.

Olive oil as diet food:

Olive oil originates from olives, the product of the olive tree. Olives are a conventional yield of the Mediterranean district. Individuals make olive oil by squeezing whole olives. Individuals utilize olive oil in cooking, beauty care products, drug, cleansers, and as a fuel for customary lights. Olive oil is originated from the Mediterranean; however, today, it is well known far and wide. In the eating regimen, individuals save olives in olive oil or salted water. They eat them entire or slashed and added to pizzas and different dishes. They can utilize olive oil a plunge for bread, for sprinkling on pasta, in cooking, or as a plate of mixed greens dressing. A few people expend it by the spoonful for therapeutic purposes.

Advantages

Additional virgin olive oil, which is the best quality oil accessible, is wealthy in cancer prevention agents, which help forestall cell harm brought about by atoms called free radicals. Free radicals are materials that the body produces in between digestion and different procedures. Cancer prevention agents kill free radicals. On the off chance that too many free radicals develop, they can cause oxidative pressure. This can prompt cell harm, and it might assume a job in the advancement of specific maladies, including particular kinds of malignant growth.

Olive oil and the cardiovascular framework

Olive oil is the primary wellspring of fat in the Mediterranean eating routine. Individuals who devour this eating routine seem to have a higher future, including a lower possibility of biting the dust from cardiovascular infections, contrasted and individuals who follow different weight control plans. A few specialists call it "the standard in preventive medication."

A recent report looked at the number of cardiovascular occasions among individuals who expended a Mediterranean eating routine, either with olive oil or nuts, or a low-fat eating regimen. Individuals who devoured the Mediterranean eating routine, regardless of whether with olive oil or nuts, had a lower occurrence of cardiovascular illness than those on the low-fat eating routine.

As indicated by the creators of one 2018 survey, the Food and Drug Administration (FDA) and the European Food Safety Authority prescribe expending around 20 grams (g) or two tablespoons (tbs) of additional virgin olive oil every day to diminish the danger of cardiovascular infection and aggravation.

Consequences of a recent report proposed that the polyphenols in additional virgin olive oil may offer security from cardiovascular sickness, atherosclerosis, stroke, mind brokenness, and malignancy. Polyphenols are a cause of cancer prevention agent.

Metabolic disorder

A metabolic disorder is a condition described by a gathering of hazard factors that expansion infection chance, including heftiness, hypertension, and high glucose levels.

Creators of a 2019 meta-examination inferred that olive oil in a Mediterranean eating routine might improve highlights of metabolic disorder, for example, irritation, glucose, triglycerides (fats in the blood), and low-thickness lipoprotein (LDL), or "terrible" cholesterol. Interestingly, it seems to build levels of high-thickness lipoprotein (HDL), or "great" cholesterol.

Wretchedness hazard and olive oil

In 2013, a rat study proposed that fixings in additional virgin olive oil may help ensure the sensory system and could be valuable for treating sadness and nervousness.

Olive oil and malignancy hazard

A few investigations have recommended that substances in olive oil may help diminish the danger of bosom malignant growth, yet not all discoveries affirm this.

As indicated by look into distributed in 2019, olive oil contains substances that may help forestall colorectal malignant growth. Lab tests have discovered proof that cell reinforcements in olive oil may help shield the body from irritation, oxidative harm, and epigenetic changes.

Alzheimer's illness

In 2016, a few researchers proposed that including additional virgin olive oil in the eating routine may help forestall Alzheimer's sickness. This might be because of its protective effect on veins in mind. Creators of a mouse study distributed in 2019 recommended that devouring oleocanthal-rich additional virgin olive oil could help moderate or stop the movement of Alzheimer's. Oleocanthal is a phenolic aggravate that happens in extra virgin olive oil.

Olive oil and the liver

A 2018 survey of research facility examines found that particles in additional virgin olive oil may help forestall or fix liver harm. The oil's MUFAs, which are predominantly oleic corrosive, and its phenolic mixes seem to help prevent aggravation, oxidative pressure, insulin obstruction, and different changes that can bring about liver harm.

Olive oil and provocative gut infection

Provocative gut infection (IBD) causes aggravation of the stomach related tract. Ulcerative colitis and Crohn's illness are kinds of IBD. A 2019 audit found that phenols in olive oil may help support intestinal insusceptibility and gut wellbeing by changing the microorganisms in the gut. This could be valuable for individuals with colitis and different kinds of IBD. The creators noticed that progressively human investigations are expected to affirm these outcomes. Discover increasingly about the Mediterranean eating routine.

Dim chocolate as diet food:

Overlook the individuals who state chocolate is garbage. Dull chocolate is stacked with supplements and studies have indicated that it is likewise useful for patching broken hearts.

Produced using the seeds of the cocoa tree, dim chocolate is perhaps the best wellspring of cancer prevention agents. Numerous examinations have demonstrated that dull chocolate can improve wellbeing and lower the danger of coronary illness among different advantages like balancing out glucose, controlling hunger, assisting with lessening yearnings and in this way encouraging weight reduction.

Be that as it may, what makes dull chocolate a super nourishment? It is cacao or cocoa bean which is stuffed with healthy synthetic concoctions like flavonoids and theobromine. When expended with some restraint, this flavorful treat has some amazing medical advantages.

Aides in diminishing cholesterol: Consumption of cocoa has been appeared to decrease levels of "awful" cholesterol (LDL) and raise levels of "good" cholesterol, conceivably bringing down the danger of cardiovascular infection. Dull chocolate is useful for skin: The flavones in dim chocolate can ensure the skin against sun harm by retaining UV and securing and increment blood stream to the surface.

It can assist you in getting more fit: YES! Chocolate can help you with shedding pounds. As indicated by neuroscientist Will Clower, a little square of good chocolate softened on the tongue 20 minutes before a feast triggers the hormones in the cerebrum that state. Completing a supper with a similar little trigger could lessen consequent nibbling. It might forestall diabetes: It sounds crazy, yet cocoa has been appeared to improve insulin affectability. So dim chocolate with some restraint may postpone or prevent the beginning of diabetes.

It can improve your state of mind: Dark chocolates cause you to feel better by animating the creation of endorphins, which is a substance in the cerebrum that expedite sentiments of delight. It additionally contains the substance serotonin, which goes about as a stimulant, subsequently causing you to feel better.

Buckwheat as diet food:

Buckwheat is a wheat crop that develops all through the United States. It is a pseudocereal as it shares numerous comparable properties to oats; however, it doesn't originate from the grass as most different oats do. Quinoa is another case of a pseudocereal.

Buckwheat is fixing in numerous ordinary nourishment items, for example, breakfast food sources, flour, and noodles. Ranchers likewise use it for animals feed. Buckwheat contains an assortment of refreshing supplements. It is a decent wellspring of protein, fibre, and stimulating complex starches.

One cup, or 168 grams (g), of broiled, cooked buckwheat groats (hulled seeds) contains the accompanying supplements:

- 5.68 g of protein
- **1.04 g of fat**
- **33.5 g of starch**
- **4.5 g of fibre**
- **148 milligrams (mg) of potassium**
- **118 mg of phosphorus**
- **86 mg of magnesium**
- **12 mg of calcium**
- 1.34 mg of iron

Buckwheat additionally contains nutrients, including:

- thiamin
- **riboflavin**
- **niacin**
- **folate**
- **nutrient K**
- nutrient B-6

The American Heart Association (AHA) suggest that at any rate, a large portion of the grains in an individual's eating routine ought to be entire grains. Entire grain nourishments contain supplements that are significant for heart wellbeing, including fibre and niacin.

A 2015 efficient survey found a connection between consumes fewer calories that were higher in entire grain nourishments and a lower danger of coronary illness. Creature considers you have discovered that buckwheat may bring down circulatory strain, which can likewise improve heart wellbeing. Individuals who follow without gluten diets may expend lower admissions of entire grains, which implies they pass up the medical advantages they give. Counting buckwheat into the eating routine as an option in contrast to whole grains that contain gluten can convey these advantages. Buckwheat is a decent wellspring of fibre. As indicated by the AHA, dietary fibre improves blood cholesterol levels, which, like this, diminishes the danger of coronary illness, diabetes, stroke, and obesity.

Improving assimilation

Buckwheat is wealthy in fibre. Dietary fibre is a kind of plant-based starch that the body can't separate during absorption. Fibre bolsters the digestion tracts in processing nourishment proficiently and assists nourishment with travelling through the stomach related tract. It might likewise have different advantages, for example, empowering weight reduction and forestalling cardiovascular infection. One cup of buckwheat additionally contains 1.58 mg of the prescribed 14 to 16 mg of niacin for grown-ups. Niacin, or nutrient B-3, is fundamental for changing over starches, fats, and proteins into vitality for the body's cells to utilize. Being a decent wellspring of fibre and niacin settles on buckwheat a proper decision for stomach related wellbeing.

Weight the board

Buckwheat is additionally a decent alternative for weight the executives. Satiety is the inclination of totality after a supper. It is a significant idea in forestalling pressure put on or advancing weight reduction. Nourishments that expansion satiety can balance long for increasingly broadened periods and may lessen the all outnumber of calories an individual expends during a day.

Buckwheat is high in protein. Research has discovered that high-protein nourishments are fundamental for weight the executives since they lead to more prominent satiety with fewer calories than different kinds of nourishment. Remembering buckwheat for a stimulating eating routine could prompt more noteworthy satiety and help with weight the board. Be that as it may, researchers should do an additional investigation into the impact of buckwheat and other entire grains to affirm this.

Overseeing diabetes

In general grain, buckwheat is a wellspring of complex sugar. This type of starch can assist individuals in dealing with their blood glucose levels. The body takes more time to separate complex sugars than straightforward carbohydrates. This hinders assimilation and assists keep with blooding sugar levels stable for more. White bread is a case of a direct sugar. As per the American Diabetes Association, entire grain nourishments are a decent wellspring of sugar. These nourishments are a fantastic wellspring of vitality and can give fibre and minerals. Creature inquire about has discovered that buckwheat positively affected insulin and blood glucose in mice with diabetes on a high-glucose diet. In any case, it is hazy whether these discoveries stretch out to people with diabetes.

Matcha Green tea as diet food:

Matcha is a sort of green tea made by taking young tea leaves and granulating them into a brilliant green powder. The powder is then sped with heated water. This is not the same as customary green tea, where the leaves are imbued in water, at that point evacuated. Drinking blended green tea "is somewhat similar to bubbling spinach, discarding the spinach and simply

181

drinking the water," says Louise Cheadle, co-writer of The Book of Matcha and co-proprietor of the tea organization tea pigs. "You will get a portion of the supplements, yet you're discarding the best piece." With matcha, you're drinking the entire tea leaves.

What are matcha tea benefits?

Matcha contains a class of cell reinforcements called catechins. Matcha is high inEGCG (epigallocatechin gallate), which is accepted to have malignant growth battlingoutcomesfor the body . Studies have connected green tea to an array of medical advantages, such as assisting with forestalling coronary illness, type 2 diabetes and malignant growth, and in any event, empowering weight reduction. Be that as it may, note that quite a bit of this exploration isn't from clinical preliminaries that show green tea causes an advantage.Matcha is even less concentrated than prepared green tea.

Turmeric as diet food:

Turmeric or Curcuma Longa is a zest mainstream in Indian curries and different dishes, yet the root holds something beyond culinary advantages. Numerous specialists consider tumeric one of the most dominant and compelling herbs. Throughout the hundreds of years and into today, it has been utilized to forestall and treat numerous infirmities. More than 10,000 distributed investigations talk about the advantages of this zest and its utilization in recuperating infections and sicknesses. Many feature that curcumin, a compound in turmeric, has more impact than some physician endorsed drugs.

Turmeric is a flavour that originates from the turmeric plant. It is usually utilized in Asian nourishment.It contains a yellow-hued substance called curcumin, which is regularly used to shading nourishments and beautifiers.

Turmeric is usually utilized for conditions including torment and aggravation, for example, osteoarthritis. It is additionally used for feed fever, melancholy, elevated cholesterol, a sort of liver sickness, and tingling. A few people use turmeric for indigestion, thinking and memory abilities, incendiary inside ailment, stress, and numerous different conditions, yet they're nothing more than trouble logical proof to help these employments.

How can it work?

Turmeric contains the concoction curcumin. Curcumin and different synthetic compounds in turmeric may diminish growing (irritation). Along these lines, turmeric may help treat conditions that include irritation.

Turmeric Gradually Increases Antioxidants in Your Body

The cell reinforcement impact of turmeric is probably the best speciality. Oxidative harm is one of the components answerable for maturing and numerous infections. Free radicals respond with natural substances in the body, which can cause hurt.

Turmeric contains curcumin, an incredible cancer prevention agent that can shield from free radicals by killing them, because of its concoction structure. Curcumin likewise invigorates cell reinforcement systems in the body.

Pecans as diet food:

Walnuts contain especially strong cell reinforcements Walnuts are rich in polyphenol cancer prevention agents, explicitly flavonoids, which have been attached to heart benefits. Truth be told, the nuts have more than double the flavonoid content found in almonds, cashews, and pistachios, and multiple times the sum in pecans. Contrasted with different nuts, walnuts likewise have the most elevated levels of gamma-tocopherols, which is a type of nutrient E and another critical cancer prevention agent. Two separate examinations have recommended that the expansion in gamma-tocopherols levels from eating a walnut luxurious eating routine forestalls the oxidation of cholesterol. Oxidized cholesterol is a hazard factor for coronary illness.

They're additionally plentiful in minerals

Walnuts are an incredible wellspring of thiamin and zinc, just as manganese and copper. One ounce (around 19 parts) supplies 60% of the Daily Value (DV) for manganese, and 40% of the DV for copper. Manganese controls glucose and is required for sound bones. This mineral additionally helps structure collagen, which gives skin its solidness and versatility. Copper helps in iron ingestion and works with iron to enable the body to frame red platelets. It likewise bolsters resistance, and assists keep with blooding vessels, nerves, and bones stable.

What's more, they're generally sweet

One ounce of walnuts contains only one gram of sugar. In any case, contrasted with different nuts, walnuts taste better. That implies they can help fulfil a sweet desiring with no or less included sugar. You can nibble on a bunch, or pair them with the organic product (walnuts work out in the right way for apples, pears, grapes, and kiwi). Toward the beginning of the day, take a stab at mixing walnuts into a smoothie; or add them to hot or cold oat, oats, a yoghurt parfait, or muesli. Trees likewise add natural sweetness and mash to exquisite dishes. Sprinkle them onto cooked veggies, entire grains, beets, spaghetti squash, fish, chicken, the fish serving of mixed greens, or entrée plates of mixed greens. (Look at this formula for Mixed Green Salad With Dried Plums and Toasted Pecans.) Or utilize hacked walnuts as a topping for hummus, soup, bean stew, pan-sears, and lettuce wraps. For a superfood treat, plunge walnut parts into softened dim chocolate and residue with ground cinnamon (yum), or use walnut margarine and slashed walnuts as the base for vitality balls, blended in with cleaved dried figs, raisins, or apples, moved oats, cinnamon, nutmeg, and ginger.

Arugula as diet food:

Arugula is a lesser realized cruciferous vegetable that gives a large number of indistinguishable advantages from different plants of a similar family, which incorporate broccoli, kale, and Brussels grows. Arugula leaves, otherwise called rocket or roquette, are delicate and scaled-down with a tart flavour. Alongside other verdant greens, arugula contains elevated levels of valuable nitrates and polyphenols.

A 2014 survey study found that high admissions of nitrate may bring down pulse, lessen the measure of oxygen required during activity, and upgrade athletic execution. This gives a top to bottom take a gander at the conceivable medical advantages of arugula, a wholesome breakdown, how to add it to the eating regimen, and conceivable wellbeing dangers connected with eating arugula.

Advantages

Eating arugula may help diminish malignant growth hazard. Eating foods grown from the ground of different types decreases the danger of numerous unfavourable wellbeing conditions because of their elevated levels of cancer prevention agents, fibre, and phytochemicals. Research has explicitly connected arugula and different cruciferous vegetables with the accompanying medical advantages:

1. Decreased malignancy hazard

While a general refreshing, vegetable-rich eating routine diminishes an individual's malignancy chance, examines have indicated that specific gatherings of vegetables can have definite anti-cancer advantages.

A 2017 meta-examination connected eating progressively cruciferous vegetables with decreased absolute malignancy chance, alongside a decrease in the whole reason mortality.

Cruciferous vegetables are a wellspring of glucosinolates, which are sulfur-containing substances. Glucosinolates might be answerable for the plants' harsh taste and their malignancy battling power. The body separates glucosinolates into a scope of advantageous mixes, including sulforaphane.

Scientists have discovered that sulforaphane can repress the chemical histone deacetylase (HDAC), which is associated with the movement of malignant growth cells. The capacity to stop HDAC proteins could make nourishments that contain sulforaphane a possibly unique piece of fatal growth treatment later on. Reports have connected weight control plans high in cruciferous vegetables with a diminished danger of bosom cancerous growth, colorectal disease, lung malignancy, prostate malignancy, and that's just the beginning. In any case, the examination is constrained, and researchers need all the more top-notch proof before affirming these advantages. Effortlessly perceived cruciferous vegetables incorporate broccoli, cauliflower, kale, cabbage, Brussels sprouts, and turnips. Less notable sorts combine arugula, bok choy, and watercress.

2. Osteoporosis anticipation

 Arugula likewise adds to an individual's day by day requirement for calcium, giving 32 milligrams (mg) per cup, going towards the DV of 1,000 mg for grown-ups.

3. Diabetes

A few audits examine have discovered that eating vegetables lessens an individual's danger of creating type 2 diabetes. A survey study from 2016 reports that verdant green vegetables are particularly useful.

One test-tube study indicated that arugula remove had antidiabetic impacts in mouse skeletal muscle cells. They created this impact by invigorating glucose take-up in the cells.

Besides, arugula and different cruciferous vegetables are a decent wellspring of fibre, which assists with directing blood glucose and may decrease insulin obstruction. High fibre nourishments cause individuals to feel more full for more, which means they can help handle indulging.

4. Heart wellbeing

Vegetable admission, explicitly cruciferous vegetables, effects affect the heart. A 2017 meta-examination reports that diets wealthy in cruciferous vegetables, servings of mixed greens, and verdant green vegetables have joined with a decreased danger of cardiovascular sickness.

Further, a recent report distributed in the Journal of the American Heart Association revealed that expending an eating regimen high in cruciferous vegetables could decrease atherosclerosis in more established ladies. Atherosclerosis is a typical condition where plaque develops in the supply routes, expanding an individual's danger of cardiovascular issues. The defensive heart impacts of these vegetables might be because of their high convergence of valuable plant mixes, including polyphenols and organosulfur blends.

Lovage as diet food:

Lovage is a plant. The root and underground stem (rhizome) are utilized to make a drug. A few people accept lovage by mouth as "water system treatment" for agony and growing (aggravation) of the lower urinary tract, for forestalling of kidney stones, and to expand the progression of pee during urinary tract diseases. Yet, there is nothing more than a bad memory relevant research to help the utilization of lovage for these or different conditions.

The little-known herb lovage is one of the leading 20 wellbeing nourishments as indicated by the writers of The Sirtfood Diet, a persuading new book about ideal sustenance for wellbeing and weight reduction.

Lovage is rich in quercetin, an intense cancer prevention agent with a variety of medical advantages.lovage was once acclaimed as a Spanish fly – adept for Valentine's Day. (The name lovage originates from 'adoration throb'; 'hurt' being the old name for parsley and nothing to do with broken hearts.)

You can utilize lovage leaves from numerous points of view: as a trimming, in servings of mixed greens or omelettes, or steamed as a side – 'stunning with cook chicken', says Hugh Fearnley-Whittingstall. In nourishments and drinks, lovage is utilized for flavouring. In fabricating; lovage is being used as a scent in cleansers and beauty care products.

How can it work?

The synthetic compounds in lovage may expand water misfortune through pee, decline fits, and help battle diseases.

Crisp lovage surrenders produce over to 1 per cent organic oil, while the dried leaf has about a portion of that sum. As far as concoction parts, the natural oil is made predominantly out of phthalides butylphthalide, sedanolide) with littler amounts of caracole (additionally found in thyme and oregano oil), eugenol and α-terpineol.

Benefits:

1.Urinary Tract Infections

A urinary tract disease or UTI can be characterized just like contamination in any piece of the urinary framework, which incorporates the kidneys, ureters, bladder and urethra.

A logical survey of 17 clinical investigations of a phytotherapeutic medicates containing lovage (just as rosemary) was distributed in 2013 and focused towards lovage as a homegrown fixing that can assist with battling microscopic organisms and lessen irritation in the urinary tract.

In a relevant article distributed the World Journal of Urology, lovage makes the rundown of herbal prescriptions for the urinary tract. The article refers to terpenoids and coumarins as the significant dynamic mixes in lovage (Leviticus officinal) root. It likewise proceeds to state that, "clinically it goes about as a more strong diuretic than parsley" and it is endorsed by the German Commission E for use in lower urinary tract diseases and urinary rock (urinary stores or stones).

For urinary issues, a tea made with a few grams of Levisticum officinal root and one cup of high temp water secured for 15–20 minutes is prescribed multiple times day by day. Another alternative is a tincture, 0.5–2 ml various times day by day.

2. Irritated Stomach

Have you at any point experienced dyspepsia? Additionally called acid reflux or upset stomach, dyspepsia is a disagreeable and fundamental wellbeing concern. In customary prescription, Levisticum officinale has been utilized for a considerable length of time to mitigate the stomach related tract, diminishing agony, swelling and gas. A few sources state the plant has additionally been generally used to treat colic and gas in kids.

3. Dysmenorrhea and Irregular Periods

For ladies, lovage might have the option to help with dysmenorrhea just as sporadic periods. As indicated by customary utilization of the herb, it can go about as a guide for ladies as an emmenagogue, or specialist that incites monthly cycle and controls its stream. This can be useful in a circumstance where menstrual cycles are deferred and unpredictable. Levisticum officinal may likewise diminish the agony related to dysmenorrhea.

Conclusion

If you need to give the Sirtfood diet a go yet you lack in time (or kitchen abilities), the organization behind the eating regimen have propelled a conveyance administration that gives you a choice to follow the arrangement, less all the cleaving.

Generally speaking, Dr Youdim would not prescribe this eating routine. There are different ways that you can decrease calorie consumption without being so prohibitive in the nourishments that you eat. The eating regimen isn't really "unfortunate" so she wouldn't alert against it if a patient discovered achievement.

If you do follow this arrangement, make sure to eat a lot of protein and change the nourishments you eat to forestall nutrient lacks. Our take? The eating regimen is inconceivably severe, and its viability has not been enough demonstrated. You're greatly improved off building up a way of life of eating an assortment of entire nourishments in the extents that suit your individual needs.

Proceed, eat more "sirtfoods," yet perhaps reconsider before really focusing on the Sirtfood Diet. Both Cording and Large man-Roth concur that plant-based, cell reinforcement stuffed "sirtfoods" can make an adequately robust expansion to your eating regimen and assist support with weighting misfortune or sound weight upkeep. In any case, concerning the eating regimen itself, there's horrible science to propose it will initiate your "thin qualities" or meaningfully affect sirtuins.

www.ingramcontent.com/pod-product-compliance
Lightning Source LLC
Chambersburg PA
CBHW060324030426
42336CB00011B/1190